Conscious Sedation,

Anesthesia, and

The JCAHO

Dean F. Smith, MD

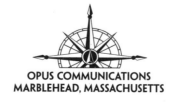

OPUS COMMUNICATIONS
MARBLEHEAD, MASSACHUSETTS

Conscious Sedation, Anesthesia, and The JCAHO is published by Opus Communications.

Copyright 1999 by Opus Communications, Inc.

All rights reserved. Printed in the United States of America. 5 4 3 2 1

ISBN 1-57839-061-3

Opus Communications provides informational resources for the health-care industry. A selected listing of our newsletters and other books is found in the back of this book. Arrangements can be made for quantity discounts.

Dean F. Smith, MD, Author
Jennifer I. Cofer, Executive Publisher
Rob Stuart, Publisher
David Beardsley, Executive Editor
Jean St. Pierre, Art Director
Cynthia Cross, Graphic Artist
Mike Mirabello, Graphic Artist
Thomas Philbrook, Cover Designer
Phyllis Lindsay, Proofreader

Advice given is general. Readers should consult professional counsel for answers to specific legal, ethical, or clinical questions. Opus Communications is not affiliated in any way with the Joint Commission on Accreditation of Healthcare Organizations.

For more information on this or other Opus Communications publications, contact:

Opus Communications
PO Box 1168
Marblehead, MA 01945
Telephone: 800/650-6787 or 781/639-1872
Fax: 800/639-8511 or 781/639-2982
E-mail: customer_service@opuscomm.com
Web site: www.opuscomm.com

Table of Contents

About the Author

Dean F. Smith, MD, is board certified in anesthesiology and pediatrics. He is in private practice in pediatric anesthesiology with Valley Anesthesiology Consultants, Ltd., in Phoenix, Arizona. Dr. Smith is the past chairman of anesthesia and the current vice president of the medical staff at St. Joseph's Hospital and Medical Center in Phoenix. He currently chairs that facility's Quality Council.

Acknowledgments

The author gratefully acknowledges the technical assistance, skills, and patience of Anna Aleksandrowicz, David Beardsley, Kim McTighe Smith, RN, Jan Magallanez, RN, Patricia Durlam, RN, John Bull, MD, Theresa Garcia, and Ginny Blossom. Thanks also to Courtney, Matt, and Mallory Smith for their patience and support.

The author also would like to thank Richard Alexander, MD, Pamela Avery, MD, Beverly Pybus, CMSC, Richard Thompson, MD, and Jack Zusman, MD, for their thoughtful reviews, suggestions, and comments. Thanks, also, to the hospitals and organizations that contributed material for this book, especially St. Joseph's Hospital and Medical Center and Catholic Healthcare West—Arizona.

Introduction

In late 1995, former White House Press Secretary James Brady was being prepared for oral surgery at an ambulatory surgery facility in Fairfax County, Virginia. Attended by both an oral surgeon and an anesthesiologist, Mr. Brady experienced cardiac arrest after receiving intravenous sedation and local anesthesia. His heart rhythms, according to media reports, ranged from dangerously low rates to ventricular fibrillation, which can be deadly. The doctors performed cardiopulmonary resuscitation and endotracheal intubation, gave resuscitative drugs, and defibrillated Mr. Brady several times.

The physicians monitored Mr. Brady throughout the resuscitation, and he apparently never suffered a lack of oxygen in his bloodstream. His condition stabilized on the way to Fairfax Hospital, where he was admitted to the intensive care unit. He recovered, having had no additional problems, and was discharged. Mr. Brady's wife, Sarah, credited the oral surgeon and the anesthesiologist with saving her husband's life.[1]

Healthcare practitioners in the United States currently perform about 25 million procedures each year involving anesthetics, and millions

---

[1] David Brown and Marylou Tousignant, "Hospital Upgrades James Brady's Condition to Fair," Washington Post, November 30, 1995, C, 3:1.

more involving sedation. In each instance, it's possible for complications like Mr. Brady's to occur. But even with a rapid increase in the use of anesthetics, anesthesia safety has improved dramatically over the last 40 years.[2]

There are a number of reasons for the decrease in anesthetic morbidity and mortality, including:

- improvements in monitoring technology, such as pulse oximetry and capnometry;
- an increase in the number of physicians who practice anesthesiology;
- better training for anesthesiologists and certified registered nurse anesthetists;
- an increase in the number of highly skilled individuals who choose to enter these fields;
- safer anesthetic agents;
- more accurate systems for delivering anesthetic agents; and
- development of and adherence to effective practice standard for perioperative care.

Nonetheless, administration of anesthesia or sedation and analgesia remain high-risk procedures. Providers cannot afford to let their vigilance wane—for the sake of patient safety and optimal patient outcomes. Also, most anesthesia or sedation and analgesia is administered

---

[2] *A comprehensive review found that anesthesia-related mortality rates fell by 50–80 percent between 1948 and 1980 (Frederick Orkin, MD, "Practice Standards: The Midas Touch or The Emperor's New Clothes?"* Anesthesiology *1989; 70: 567-71). Also, among 319,000 consecutive patients who were either healthy or had a mild systemic disease (classified by the American Society of Anesthesiologists as Physical Status I and II) and who received anesthesia at the Harvard-affiliated hospitals, there were no major preventable intraoperative injuries (John H. Eichhorn, MD, "Prevention of Intraoperative Anesthesia Accidents and Related Severe Injury Through Safety Monitoring,"* Anesthesiology *1989; 70: 572-7).*

in facilities that are accredited by the Joint Commission on Accreditation of Healthcare Organizations (JCAHO). The information in this book is designed to help you protect patients and comply with the JCAHO standards as they relate to anesthesia.

Chapter 1 discusses when the JCAHO's anesthesia standards apply to sedation cases and gives basic compliance recommendations.

Chapter 2 discusses the JCAHO's anesthesia-related standards in more detail, providing all the compliance information you'll need, and includes tables that identify relevant standards by number.

Chapter 3 addresses credentialing and privileging in the context of conscious sedation and anesthesia care, including an overview of the requirements of the JCAHO and of professional organizations that certify anesthesia providers.

Chapter 4 discusses preparation for a JCAHO survey on the anesthesia standards, concluding with a case study on how St. Joseph's Hospital and Medical Center in Phoenix, Arizona, implemented changes in its anesthesia practice to satisfy JCAHO requirements.

Chapter 5 explains how to develop a quality monitoring program for anesthesia that's based on the continuous quality improvement (CQI) model.

The appendices include sample policies and guidelines from the American Society of Anesthesiologists, and material to help you educate patients and their families about anesthesia care.

This publication is designed to help you promote safe and effective use of anesthesia, analgesia, and sedation, while also preparing your facility for key elements of its next JCAHO survey.

Anesthesia Versus Sedation

A focus on improving patient safety in anesthesia care—which began in earnest in the early 1980s with endeavors such as the Anesthesia Patient Safety Foundation—has made administration of anesthetics, sedatives, and analgesics one of the safest high-risk procedures in medicine. It has also made compliance with the JCAHO's standards for anesthesia care among the least troubling accreditation issues, with one exception: procedures that involve sedation and analgesia, which the JCAHO terms conscious sedation.[1] In these instances, compliance with the anesthesia standards has been more problematic, largely because the standards don't always apply and because many health-care facilities have trouble determining when they do.

Not all JCAHO surveyors will address the issue of conscious sedation. But, because it is a source of confusion and noncompliance, don't be surprised if the topic comes up during your next survey. A poll of more

---

[1]A significant portion of the anesthesia community prefers the phrase "sedation and analgesia," but the JCAHO still uses "conscious sedation." Since this book focuses on accreditation-related issues, and since it is designed primarily for a non-clinical audience, the author will often use the JCAHO's preferred term, "conscious sedation." However, the author acknowledges that the term may be somewhat out of date and stresses that it should be viewed as synonymous with "sedation and analgesia."

than 100 hospitals surveyed in 1996 suggests that questions on conscious sedation were common that year:

- JCAHO surveyors asked 76 percent of the hospitals about their policies on conscious sedation.
- They asked 81 percent of respondents to tell them who performs pre-operative assessments.
- Surveyors asked 76 percent of the hospitals to identify who in the organization is allowed to administer conscious sedation.[2]

Ninety-three hospitals surveyed during the first three quarters of 1998 revealed the following:

- Surveyors asked about conscious sedation policies during 58 percent of the surveys.
- They asked about conscious sedation privileges in 48 percent of the surveys.
- They asked about pre-operative assessments 47 percent of the time.[3]

Finally, 16 hospitals that underwent a JCAHO survey in the first quarter of 1999 reported the following:

- JCAHO surveyors asked 69 percent of them about their policies on conscious sedation.
- They asked 63 percent of respondents to identify who in the organization is allowed to administer conscious sedation.

---

[2] *Briefings on JCAHO Post-JCAHO–Survey Questionnaire, Opus Communications (Marblehead, MA), 4th Quarter, 1996.*

[3] *Opus Communications, "What's happening during Joint Commission Surveys: Third quarter 1998," A special report from:* Briefings on JCAHO, *October 1999*

- Surveyors asked 44 percent of the hospitals to tell them who performs pre-operative assessments.
- They asked 56 percent of the hospitals about anesthesia pre-assessments.[4]

This book will prepare your organization to respond to such questions, and it will help you design policies and procedures for conscious sedation that improve patient safety and satisfy the expectations of JCAHO surveyors.

When do the JCAHO standards on anesthesia apply?

Physicians and employees at some facilities believe that the delineated clinical privileges of the practitioner administering conscious sedation determines whether the anesthesia standards apply. Others think the determining factor is the type of drug(s) in use. These are common misconceptions. The anesthesia standards apply when patients receive general or major regional anesthesia (e.g., spinal or epidural anesthesia), or when they receive sedatives or analgesics by any route, for any purpose, or in any setting that "may be reasonably expected to result in the loss of protective reflexes—an inability to handle secretions without aspiration or to maintain a patent airway independently" (*CAMH*, TX–15).

Patients who receive local anesthesia, regional anesthesia, or sedation (with or without analgesia) usually do not lose their ability to breathe or to handle airway secretions (see Exhibit 1). Occasionally, however, there are factors that cause them to do so—at which point they have

---

[4] *Opus Communications, "What's happening during Joint Commission surveys: First quarter 1999," A special report from:* Briefings on JCAHO, *April 1999.*

> **Exhibit 1**
>
> # Why use sedation?
>
> Because patients who receive conscious sedation usually retain their protective reflexes, and because recovery from sedation is commonly more rapid and less likely to have side effects associated with anesthesia (nausea, vomiting, etc.), practitioners often prefer sedating patients to anesthetizing them. This is especially true for many operative procedures that take place in ambulatory centers and for diagnostic and invasive procedures, including:
>
> - biopsies,
> - laceration repairs,
> - orthopedic or podiatric procedures,
> - dental or oral surgery procedures,
> - gastrointestinal endoscopies,
> - bronchoscopies,
> - radiographic studies, and
> - cardiac catheterizations.
>
> Practitioners also find sedation preferable to anesthesia when they need patients to respond to verbal or tactile stimulation during a procedure. In these instances, some sedatives and analgesics make it easier for practitioners to complete procedures because they alleviate patient pain and anxiety—which, in turn, minimizes undesirable patient movement. Unlike anesthesia, however, these medications may not eliminate a patient's ability to interact with the practitioner and to function, as needed, during a procedure.

moved beyond sedation into the realm of anesthesia. In these instances, the anesthesia standards apply in full.

Key requirements of the JCAHO standards

Chapter two examines all the JCAHO standards relevant to anesthesia care, discussing compliance in a context that includes instances when sedated patients lose their protective reflexes. However, a few of those standards are particularly relevant to this chapter's discussion of the "gray area" where conscious sedation and anesthesia overlap. It's worth discussing the requirements of those standards here.

Patient assessments

Standards in the "Care of Patients (TX)" chapter of the JCAHO's *Comprehensive Accreditation Manual for Hospitals* (*CAMH*) and in the chapter titled "Assessment of Patients (PE)" require hospitals to evaluate all patients before they undergo a procedure involving anesthesia—an evaluation that is known as a "pre-anesthetic assessment." From an accreditation standpoint, the implications of this requirement clearly illustrate why organizations must have criteria for deciding when conscious sedation is likely to become anesthesia (that is, when sedated patients have a reasonable chance of losing their protective reflexes and the ability to breathe on their own). Once that happens, it's too late to perform a pre-anesthetic assessment. The best way to ensure effective compliance with this JCAHO requirement is to develop and enforce a sedation policy that requires practitioners to treat sedation as anesthesia any time the use of sedatives or analgesics could possibly lead to loss of protective reflexes.

Clearly, it is impossible for physicians and other practitioners to predict every instance in which airway reflexes are lost and sedation becomes anesthesia—too many variables come into play, including:

- the patient's age and health status;
- the drug dosage and method of administration;
- the additive effects of sedatives and/or analgesics used in combination; and
- the additive effects of other drugs the patient is taking.

The JCAHO recognizes this variability. Surveyors won't expect you to forecast all crossovers; nor will they perform a comprehensive review of your medical records looking for all instances when sedated patients lost their protective reflexes. Rather, they'll want assurances, backed by documented evidence, that your criteria for evaluating the risks and likely effects of sedation allow you to identify instances that "may be *reasonably* expected to result in the loss of protective reflexes" (*CAMH*, TX-15, emphasis added).

The more data-driven your criteria for assessing sedation cases are, the better off you're likely to be during a JCAHO survey. The JCAHO's performance improvement (PI) standards list medication use—which includes use of sedatives, analgesics, and anesthetics—among the six high-risk, high-volume, problem-prone processes that hospitals must monitor (*CAMH*, PI-11). Since several variables affect the way patients respond to sedatives and analgesics, and because reactions to these medications can be severe, organizations should consider tracking and evaluating instances when patients receiving sedation lose their protective airway reflexes. The data might make administration of conscious sedation safer (a key goal of the JCAHO anesthesia standards) by identifying trends that help you hone your assessment criteria for sedation patients; they're likely to assist you with JCAHO compliance by helping practitioners better predict when sedation should be treated as anesthesia.

Comparable levels of care

A key standard in the "Leadership (LD)" chapter of the *CAMH* requires organizations to provide patients with a comparable level of care—regardless of the treatment setting, and no matter who provides that care. In the context of this chapter, this requirements means organizations must subject practitioners to the same policies, procedures, and standards of care for conscious sedation regardless of whether those practitioners provide the services in an inpatient operating room, an ambulatory surgical center, an examination room, or anywhere else within an organization's facilities. This has become an increasingly important requirement since the changing economics of healthcare began to trigger a wave of facility mergers and the development of multi-setting health systems—trends that have increased the range of treatment settings that exist within many organizations.

Given this mandate for a comparable level of care, organizations that are designing a performance improvement program for conscious sedation should consider tracking adverse sedation outcomes by treatment setting and practitioner type. To maximize patient safety and satisfy JCAHO surveyors, organizations need to ensure that all practitioners who are allowed to administer sedatives, analgesics, and anesthetics do so with equal skill and precision—whether they are anesthesiologists, other physicians with appropriate privileges, or certified registered nurse anesthetists (CRNAs). If performance data reveal quality gaps among practitioner types, or if they suggest that quality varies according to the treatment setting, the organization may need to revise its privileging criteria (see Chapter 3) and sedation policies.

Compliance basics

The JCAHO's *Comprehensive Accreditation Manual for Hospitals (CAMH)* outlines hundreds of standards, all of which serve as fodder for surveyor questions. Given that, it's easy to see how organizations get bogged down in minutiae as they prepare for a survey. However, it's possible to focus so closely on details that you ignore the broader intent of the JCAHO standards:

> The standards are simply articulations of the expectation that organizations will do the "right things right." And when that happens, the likelihood of bad outcomes is minimized and the potential for good outcomes is optimized (*CAMH*, Update 1, February 1998, "Foreword," FW–1).

It's often more useful and effective to prepare for a JCAHO survey by stepping back from the standards and asking everyone in the organization to answer one basic question: If I were the patient, what would I want from the person performing my job? We'll examine this question as it pertains to conscious sedation in Chapter 2, but for now it's worth noting that answers you'll receive usually generate a list of objectives similar to those laid out in the JCAHO standards. If organizations can honestly say their written policies and procedures promote a level of treatment consistent with those objectives, and if they have data documenting that performance and quality of care consistently meet those objectives, they're likely to satisfy the JCAHO.

That said, there are some basic steps organizations should take to demonstrate to JCAHO surveyors that they're prepared for instances when sedation becomes anesthesia. They need to have adequate, clearly defined criteria for identifying patients receiving sedation who are reasonably likely to lose the ability to breathe on their own and handle airway secretions. And, when a patient fits those criteria, they need to document that practitioners comply with the anesthesia standards. They should also consider developing a sedation policy (see the sample policies in Appendix A)—keeping in mind that JCAHO standards don't require a policy, but if organizations develop one, surveyors will hold them to it.[5] This policy should:

- define minimal standards of care for patients not expected to lose protective reflexes;
- include requirements for patient monitoring, personnel, and equipment;
- delineate additional requirements regarding staffing, monitoring, equipment availability, and patient evaluation and care (before, during, and after the procedure) when patients have a reasonable chance of losing their protective reflexes; and
- be consistent with state and federal law and with the facility's mission and strategic plan.[6]

Remember: The nature of the procedure, the classification of drug(s) used, and the qualifications or privileges of the practitioner administering those drugs do not determine whether the JCAHO's anesthesia

---

[5] If medical and hospital staffs don't comply with internal policies, or if hospital and physician leaders don't enforce internal policies, JCAHO surveyors will issue a Type I Recommendation—regardless of whether the JCAHO requires development of the policy in question.

[6] See also: American Society of Anesthesiologists, "Guidelines for Sedation and Analgesia by Non-Anesthesiologists," Anesthesiology 84 (1996): 459-71.

standards apply. The determining factor is the potential for a patient to lose his or her protective reflexes.

The JCAHO's Anesthesia-Related Standards

Anesthesia: The administration to an individual, in any setting, for any purpose, by any route (general, spinal, or other) of major regional anesthesia or sedation (with or without analgesia) for which there is a reasonable expectation that, in the manner used, the analgesia or sedation will result in the loss of protective reflexes (CAMH, GL-3, August 1998 update).

The link between safety, quality, and compliance

Complying with JCAHO standards and maintaining JCAHO accreditation can be challenging, time consuming, and frustrating. It's not uncommon to hear members of hospital and medical staffs complain that the time they spend dealing with compliance issues and survey preparation takes away from their top priority: caring for patients. In some instances they're just blowing off steam, but in others they've lost sight of an important fact: The JCAHO standards are designed to promote safe, effective patient care. Viewed in this light, compliance might not become less arduous, but it will come to seem less like an irrelevant distraction. This view can also form the foundation for a powerful and effective approach to survey preparation.

Pretend you are the patient

Once organizations begin to view the JCAHO standards as a vehicle for maintaining and improving quality of care and patient safety, they're likely to spend less time reading the fine print in their JCAHO standards manual and more time talking about what's best for patients. Survey coordinators and hospital and physician leaders can lead this shift by focusing survey preparation on a basic question: "If each of us were being treated here, what would we want from this organization and its caregivers?"

To assess compliance with the anesthesia standards, an organization's survey coordinator should ask leaders from anesthesiology a version of the same question: "If we were admitted to this hospital for an operation or some other procedure that involves anesthesia or sedation, what would we expect of the people responsible for that anesthesia or sedation?" The answers usually sound something like this:

- Pick the safest, most effective anesthetics or sedatives.
- Know how to administer them properly.
- Know the contraindications and side effects associated with those medications.
- Learn something about my past experiences with anesthesia or sedation ahead of time.
- Tell me what to expect.
- Allow me ample opportunity to ask questions.
- Answer my questions honestly and with authority.
- Know how I'm doing at all times during the procedure.
- Don't just rush off to the next patient and procedure; make sure the practitioners and nurses monitoring my recovery have the information they need to do a good job.
- Do all of the above whether I'm to be sedated or anesthetized.

Once you've brainstormed as many responses as possible, compare your answers with the compliance requirements discussed below. You'll probably find that you have addressed most of the major issues. Next, ask yourselves whether your current policies, procedures, and treatment systems are consistent with the responses you generated, and whether staff implement those policies, procedures, and systems effectively. If the answer to both questions is yes, you should be in good survey shape. Furthermore, if JCAHO surveyors think otherwise, you should have solid grounds for appealing Type I recommendations. If the answer to either question is no, use your responses and the guidance provided in this chapter to make the necessary changes to your policies, procedures, and systems.

What standards apply to anesthesia care?

The JCAHO standards governing anesthesia and conscious sedation (procedures during which sedated patients have a reasonable chance of losing their protective reflexes) are designed to protect patient safety and promote quality care in all settings where patients receive anesthetics, sedatives, and/or analgesics. The largest concentration of standards related to anesthesia care occurs in the "Care of Patients (TX)" chapter of the JCAHO's *Comprehensive Accreditation Manual for Hospitals (CAMH)*—specifically, standards TX.2–TX.2.4.1. However, healthcare facilities also will find standards that have direct or indirect implications for anesthesia care in the following *CAMH* chapters:

- Patient Rights and Organization Ethics (RI)
- Assessment of Patients (PE)
- Patient and Family Education (PF)
- Continuum of Care (CC)

- Improving Organization Performance (PI)
- Leadership (LD)
- Management of the Environment of Care (EC)
- Management of Human Resources (HR)
- Management of Information (IM)
- Surveillance, Prevention, and Control of Infection (IC)
- Medical Staff (MS)

Because the JCAHO includes relevant standards in so many *CAMH* chapters, some hospitals find it difficult to educate caregivers and monitor compliance. This chapter is meant to assist them by providing a comprehensive overview of the JCAHO's requirements.

Often, this chapter will make reference to anesthesia and conscious sedation. In those cases, the term conscious sedation refers to instances in which patients receiving sedatives or analgesics risk losing the reflexes that allow them to breathe and maintain an airway independently—the factor that determines whether the JCAHO anesthesia standards apply to sedation (see Chapter 1). Any time the term "anesthesia" appears on its own, readers should consider it a blanket reference that encompasses conscious sedation, wherein there is a reasonable chance of loss of protective airway reflexes. The term conscious sedation is also interchangeable with "sedation and analgesia."

The anesthesia standards and tips on compliance

Having adequate policy and procedure documents in place is only half the battle during a JCAHO survey. During interview sessions and visits to patient care areas, surveyors will question hospital staff and physicians to gauge how effectively they implement and understand your policies, procedures, and standards of care. The following list gives you a taste of the questions surveyors might ask:

- What are your criteria for determining when patients who receive sedatives or analgesics have a reasonable chance of losing their protective reflexes?
- How do you assess patients before they receive anesthesia or sedation that could cause them to lose their protective reflexes? Who assesses these patients?
- Where and when do practitioners responsible for administering anesthesia meet their patients?
- How does the facility coordinate anesthesia services with surgical and nursing services?
- Is anesthesia or conscious sedation ever administered outside the operating room? Where?
- Who monitors patients receiving anesthesia and sedation outside the operating room? How is that monitoring accomplished?
- What are the criteria for discharging patients from the post-anesthesia care unit?
- Does your facility track adverse events and outcomes in patients receiving anesthesia and conscious sedation?
- How do you ensure that only qualified practitioners administer or supervise anesthesia and conscious sedation services?

The following sections should help you prepare hospital staff and physicians to answer these and other questions by explaining the

JCAHO's standards and offering compliance advice. A grid at the beginning of each section identifies the standards being addressed (the standard numbers are current as of mid-1999). However, to avoid repetition and to promote a multidisciplinary approach to anesthesia care, there is not a section for each standard—nor are the sections organized by *CAMH* chapter. This discussion addresses the goals, expectations, and themes that run throughout the standards and across different *CAMH* chapters. Facilities where policies, procedures, and caregiver performance are consistent with the treatment objectives and activities discussed here should be well prepared for a JCAHO survey.

Informed consent for anesthesia and sedation

Relevant standards	
RI.1.2 & RI.1.2.1	TX.2.2
RI.1.2.1.1–RI.1.2.1.5	TX.5.2–TX.5.2.2
RI.1.2.2	

One aspect of providing quality care involves ensuring that patients understand and agree to the care they receive. Before patients receive anesthesia or conscious sedation, therefore, they or surrogate decision-makers (e.g., a parent or other relative, guardian, or authorized acquaintance) must authorize its use—a process known as providing informed consent. To ensure that a patient or authorized decision maker grants consent that is truly informed, practitioners should discuss the benefits, risks, possible complications of, and alternatives to the procedure in question. In the case of anesthesia or conscious sedation, that means securing consent after having thoroughly explained:

- the expected results of the procedure,
- potential complications,

- the probability of a successful outcome, and
- treatment alternatives (e.g., use of regional anesthesia rather than general anesthesia, etc.).

Practitioners must also explain the need for, risks of, and alternatives to the use of blood or blood products, should the patient require this type of treatment. Because, in many institutions, blood and blood products are most often administered by an anesthesiologist during the perioperative period, responsibility for informing patients and obtaining consent for this therapy may involve members of the anesthesia care team. To fully meet JCAHO requirements and limit liability in this area, practitioners should document their efforts to inform patients or decision-makers and their receipt of informed consent.

Healthcare facilities should encourage immediate family members to share in decisions regarding a patient's treatment, and there are times when involvement is mandatory. Parents or guardians, for instance, must be involved in decisions affecting the care of minors, including decisions regarding the use of anesthesia or conscious sedation. However, family members are not authorized to interfere with an adult's right to make healthcare-related decisions

Healthcare facilities also must help patients appoint surrogate decision-makers when physical or mental limitations prevent those patients from granting informed consent or making treatment-related decisions. The JCAHO defines "surrogate decision-maker" as "someone appointed to act on behalf of another...when an individual is without capacity or has given permission to involve others" (*CAMH*, August 1998 update, GL-24). This definition implies that such decision-makers can be family members, guardians, adult-aged friends, or anyone else whom patients appropriately authorize to act on their behalf.

Facilities, physicians, and other caregivers must also respect and protect the rights of patients participating in clinical studies. They must ensure that these patients have been informed of the potential benefits, risks, and alternatives to participation and take part in the study willingly. They must ensure that the patients know what procedures are involved, including use of anesthesia or sedation. Healthcare facilities must have a written policy outlining acceptable procedures for informing patients on these counts and securing consent. In addition, practitioners must document their efforts to inform patients and secure consent.

Compliance tips
A facility can begin to demonstrate compliance with informed consent requirements for anesthesia or conscious sedation by developing a policy that outlines acceptable means for securing informed consent and includes the following requirements:

- The practitioner who administers anesthesia or conscious sedation obtains informed consent. This practitioner should be either a licensed independent practitioner (LIP) with appropriate clinical privileges or a supervised practitioner allowed by law and the facility to sedate or anesthetize patients.

- The practitioner discusses the use of anesthesia or conscious sedation with the patient or the patient's surrogate decision-maker(s), addressing, among other things:

– the anesthesia plan;

– possible side effects and complications;

– implications of not administering the anesthesia or sedation; and

– alternatives to the planned use of anesthesia or conscious sedation.

The policy should also explain how the facility seeks to overcome disabilities, language barriers, and other factors that may affect a patient's ability to understand a procedure and provide informed consent. Such a policy might, for example, state that the facility provides translators and/or language-appropriate handouts, audio tapes, or video tapes for patients and decision-makers who don't speak English.

Facilities must also ensure that practitioners comply with the informed consent policy, and that the practitioners document their compliance in patients' medical records. During medical record reviews, JCAHO surveyors will look for the following:

- evidence of an adequate discussion between an authorized practitioner and the patient or surrogate decision-maker;
- evidence that the patient or surrogate decision-maker acknowledges understanding the relevant risks of, likely benefits and outcomes of, and reasonable alternatives to the planned procedure; and
- evidence that the patient granted informed consent for the procedure and, in the case of anesthesia or conscious sedation, the anesthesia plan.

Practitioners must make every effort to obtain informed consent from a patient or authorized surrogate decision-maker. If, in emergencies, that is not possible—that is, if a patient needs emergency care, is unable to communicate, and a surrogate decision-maker is unavailable—practitioners can provide care, but they must document the situation by clearly describing the circumstances in the patient's medical record.

Preanesthetic assessments and anesthesia planning

Relevant standards	
LD.1.3.4	TX.1 & TX.1.2
LD.1.6	TX.2 & TX.2.1
MS.6.2.1	TX.5–TX.5.1.5
PE.1.6–PE.1.6.1.1	TX.5.3
PE.1.7–PE.1.7.4	

Because anesthesia and sedation place patients at considerable risk—and because patients may respond differently to anesthetics, sedatives, and analgesics—careful planning is a key part of quality anesthesia care. Preanesthesia assessments are an important part of that planning process, and the JCAHO requires them for all procedures involving anesthesia.[1] (Remember: The JCAHO's definition of "anesthesia" goes beyond the administration of general, regional, or local anesthetics to include use of sedatives and/or analgesics that have a reasonable

---

[1] In an emergency, when there is no time to perform and document a history and physical examination, the JCAHO requires only that the patient's record include a description of the circumstances and the practitioner's preoperative diagnosis.

chance of causing patients to lose their protective reflexes.) These assessments help practitioners:

- select the most effective drug or combination of drugs with which to anesthetize or sedate patients;
- plan the administration of anesthetics or sedatives;
- administer those drugs safely; and
- interpret data obtained during patient monitoring.

An effective preanesthetic assessment reduces the chances of morbidity or mortality caused by complications from anesthesia or sedation. It should include the following elements:

- an assessment of the patient's potential for loss of protective reflexes, and a plan for how the anesthesia care team will react to such a situation;
- an interview with the patient and/or the patient's legal guardian or surrogate decision-maker, which includes a review of the patient's medical history and a focused physical examination[2] (see Figure 2.1); and
- orders for diagnostic tests, including: blood work, radiographic studies, an electrocardiogram, and pulmonary functions studies—if the history and physical examination suggest they are necessary. Results of these tests must appear in the patient's medical record.

---

[2] *If a practitioner performed a history and physical examination (H&P) on the patient within 30 days of the patient's date of admission, that H&P may be used during the preanesthetic assessment, "provided durable, legible copies (or originals) of the report are in the patient's record and any significant changes in the patient's condition since the report are recorded at the time of admission" (CAMH, PE-9).*

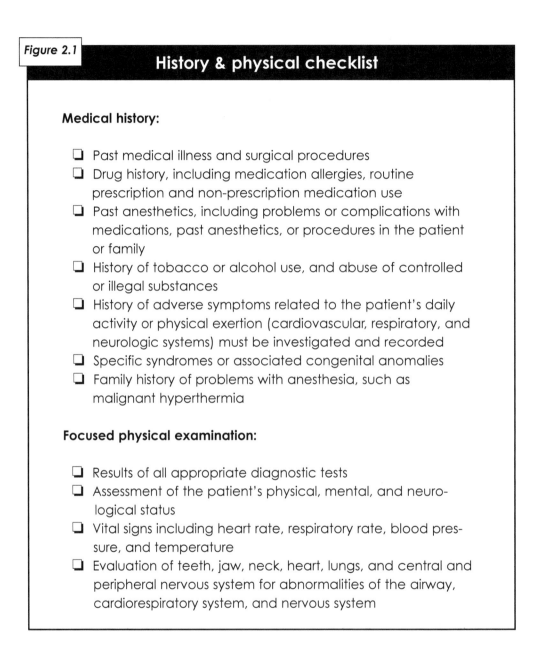

Figure 2.1

History & physical checklist

Medical history:

❑ Past medical illness and surgical procedures
❑ Drug history, including medication allergies, routine prescription and non-prescription medication use
❑ Past anesthetics, including problems or complications with medications, past anesthetics, or procedures in the patient or family
❑ History of tobacco or alcohol use, and abuse of controlled or illegal substances
❑ History of adverse symptoms related to the patient's daily activity or physical exertion (cardiovascular, respiratory, and neurologic systems) must be investigated and recorded
❑ Specific syndromes or associated congenital anomalies
❑ Family history of problems with anesthesia, such as malignant hyperthermia

Focused physical examination:

❑ Results of all appropriate diagnostic tests
❑ Assessment of the patient's physical, mental, and neuro-logical status
❑ Vital signs including heart rate, respiratory rate, blood pres-sure, and temperature
❑ Evaluation of teeth, jaw, neck, heart, lungs, and central and peripheral nervous system for abnormalities of the airway, cardiorespiratory system, and nervous system

JCAHO surveyors will assess your compliance with assessment require-ments by interviewing physicians and other relevant caregivers, and by reviewing a sample of medical records for patients who received anes-thesia and/or sedation. The practitioner who administers the anesthesia or sedation does not have to be the one who records notes on the pre-anesthetic assessment and anesthesia plan in the patient's chart, but that chart should include the following preoperative information:

- the patient's anesthesia classification code (see Figure 2.2), which helps a practitioner identify risks to the patient, appropriate drug(s), monitoring methods, and clinical monitoring parameters;
- the type of anesthesia care to be delivered: general, regional, or monitored anesthesia care;[3]

Figure 2.2

ASA physical status classification

P1—A normal, healthy patient
P2—A patient with mild systemic disease
P3—A patient with severe systemic disease
P4—A patient with severe systemic disease that is a constant threat to life
P5—A moribund patient who is not expected to survive without the operation
P6—A declared brain-dead patient whose organs are being removed for donor purposes

© 1999, American Society of Anesthesiologists, 520 N. Northwest Highway, Park Ridge, IL 60068. Reprinted by permission.

---

[3] "Monitored anesthesia care is a specific anesthesia service in which an anesthesiologist has been [asked] to participate in the care of a patient undergoing a diagnostic or therapeutic procedure. Monitored anesthesia care includes all aspects of anesthesia care—a preprocedure visit, intraoperative care, and postprocedure management" (American Society of Anesthesiologists 1999 Directory of Members, "Position on Monitored Anesthesia Care," Washington, DC: ASA, 1999, 481). The ASA position statement goes on to say that the services provided during monitored anesthesia care include monitoring of vital signs and airway management, diagnosis and treatment of problems occurring during the procedure, administration of medications to enhance patient comfort and safety, and provision of other services as needed. It acknowledges that monitored anesthesia care refers to clinical situations in which patients may or may not lose consciousness or normal protective reflexes.

- plans or orders for additional preprocedure diagnostic data, if needed, and the results of diagnostic tests performed to obtain that data;
- a practitioner's preoperative diagnosis; and
- a plan, developed prior to the procedure, for nursing care during and after administration of anesthesia or conscious sedation.

The JCAHO requires hospitals to administer anesthesia for obstetric and emergency surgical services within 30 minutes of the attending physician determining that anesthesia is necessary. The JCAHO also requires facilities to provide anesthesia for other procedures within a "reasonable time frame" after the preanesthetic assessment—leaving it up to the organization to decide what constitutes a reasonable time frame. Just before administration of the anesthesia or sedation, patients must be reassessed. This final preanesthetic assessment, which usually includes an evaluation of the patient's blood pressure, heart rate, electrocardiogram, and blood oxygenation (via pulse oximetry), must be documented.

Compliance tips

A facility's written policies and procedures are a key element of compliance with the JCAHO requirements regarding preanesthetic assessments and anesthesia planning. JCAHO surveyors will expect you to have written documents requiring practitioners to fulfill the minimum requirements for preanesthesia care that are outlined above. Furthermore, they'll expect these policies—and your enforcement of them—to apply equally to all treatment settings within your organization. As was discussed in Chapter 1, JCAHO standards require all practitioners within a single organization to provide a comparable level of care, regardless of the treatment setting; since the development of health systems and networks has made it more common for organizations to have a number of treatment settings where patients receive anesthesia and other procedures, JCAHO surveyors carefully gauge quality and performance across settings.

Surveyors assess the performance of caregivers and the quality of care provided in your organization in two basic ways: 1) by interviewing physicians and staff, and 2) by reviewing caregiver documentation in patient medical records. As you prepare for a survey, ensure that relevant caregivers can describe their roles and responsibilities in preanesthesia care, as outlined in your policies and procedures. You should also periodically audit chart documentation to ensure it indicates that practitioners consistently provide safe, high quality preanesthesia care, as defined by your policies, and that they document the provision of that care clearly and adequately. Because documentation at this stage of anesthesia care gets recorded on a number of different documents, facilities should consider creating a checklist to track it all.

Although it is not required by the JCAHO, facilities should consider incorporating relevant elements the American Society for Anesthesiologists' "Guidelines for Patient Care in Anesthesiology" (see page 157) and all elements of ASA's "Basic Standards for Preanesthesia Care" (see page 165) into documents that formalize their policies and procedures for preanesthesia assessment and planning. The guidelines in these ASA documents are consistent with many of the JCAHO's preanesthesia requirements and can help improve the quality and safety of anesthesia care.

Intraoperative anesthesia care

R e l e v a n t   s t a n d a r d s

TX.2.3	LD.1.3.2
PE.1.7.3	LD.2.7
IM.7.3	LD.2.9

The Brady case outlined in the introduction shows that a patient doesn't need to be receiving general anesthesia for monitoring to be critical to an optimal outcome. Like patients receiving general anesthesia, sedated patients might lose the ability to communicate, which means physiologic monitoring may be the only means of determining their well-being. Monitoring allows practitioners to evaluate the effects of the medication and the procedure on the patient and intervene in emergencies (the ventricular fibrillation experienced by Brady, for example, or sudden loss of protective reflexes and the ability to maintain an airway).

An authorized practitioner must monitor the heart and respiratory rates, electrocardiogram, blood pressure, and oxygenation of all patients receiving anesthesia or conscious sedation. Whether additional monitoring is necessary depends on the results of the preanesthesia assessment, the final assessment made before the procedure begins, the nature of that procedure, and the anesthetics or sedatives slated for use. All physiological data collected during the procedure must be documented in the patient's medical record.

Organizations should consider incorporating the ASA's "Standards for Basic Anesthetic Monitoring" (see page 151) into policy and procedure documents that govern intraoperative anesthesia care. In general these documents should:

- outline appropriate monitoring methods and procedures;
- identify criteria for determining which methods and procedures to use; and
- detail minimum requirements regarding documentation of monitoring data (e.g., time intervals for documenting, specificity of documentation, etc.).

Compliance tips

As with most standards, JCAHO surveyors assess compliance with intraoperative anesthesia requirements by interviewing physicians and staff, reviewing policy and procedure documents, and auditing medical record documentation. Prior to your next survey, ensure that relevant caregivers understand and can explain their roles and responsibilities during intraoperative anesthesia care. You should also review and, if necessary, revise your policies and procedures to ensure they address the minimum requirements outlined above. And, you should audit a representative sample of medical records to ensure that the anesthesia records in them document the following information for all relevant procedures:

- patient's vital signs at regular, appropriate intervals;
- the dosage of all drugs given and the time of administration;
- all fluids a patient received, including blood and blood products;
- an estimate of the volume of blood and other fluids lost by the patient;
- the method for administering anesthetics, sedatives, and/or analgesics;
- any unusual events or complications; and
- the status of the patient at the conclusion of a procedure involving anesthesia or conscious sedation.

Postanesthesia care

Relevant standards

PE.1.7.4	IM.7.3.3
TX.2.4 & TX.2.4.1	IM.7.3.4 & IM.7.3.4.1
TX.5.4	IM.7.3.5

At the end of a procedure involving anesthesia or sedation, patients usually go to a designated postanesthesia care unit (PACU)—although some go to intensive care. In the PACU, a caregiver is assigned to monitor the patient continuously and implement an LIP's orders for postanesthesia care—notifying the appropriate LIP(s) of changes for better or worse in the patient's condition and documenting information regarding:

- fluids, including blood or blood products, that the patient received or lost (i.e., the amounts received or lost and the resulting effects);
- medications administered; and
- the patient's physiological and mental status, including:
  - blood pressure, heart rate, respiratory rate, and blood oxygenation;
  - body temperature;
  - level of consciousness;
  - circulation (perfusion of tissues);
  - condition of dressings (if relevant);
  - types of drains (e.g., chest tube) and the nature and quantity of drainage;

– condition of intravenous site(s), type and amount of solutions (medication, blood and blood products, other fluids) being infused, and their effects;

– changes in the patient's general appearance (e.g., edema, rashes, etc.);

– diaphoresis (perspiration);

– discomfort, restlessness, or apprehension; and

– complications or unexpected developments.

Depending on the nature of the procedure and the type of anesthesia or sedation used, the PACU caregiver should monitor and document other things—as required by facility policy or ordered by an LIP. Following spinal anesthesia, for example, caregivers monitor and document the patient's ability to move his or her lower extremities.

An LIP must evaluate patients before they leave the PACU and/or the patients must meet discharge criteria that have been approved by the facility's medical staff. These criteria should include:

• stable blood pressure, heart rate, and respiratory rate;
• clearly defined level of consciousness;
• no excessive bleeding; and
• no evidence of other physiological instability.

The medical record must include the name of the LIP responsible for discharging a patient and show that the patient met the facility's discharge criteria. If the patient is sent directly home from the PACU—rather than being transferred to another care setting—he or she must be accompanied by an adult.

Compliance tips

Facilities must have a policy that governs patient care during the postanesthesia period. They should consider using ASA's "Standards for Postanesthesia Care" (see page 161) when developing that policy. Their policy must apply to all patients who receive general anesthesia, major regional anesthesia, or sedation that could result in loss of protective reflexes. In general, the policy should require:

- PACUs to have specified medical and nursing leadership;
- comparable levels of care in PACUs throughout an organization or facility; and
- compliance with identical discharge criteria in PACUs through-out the organization or facility.

The policy must also outline requirements for monitoring of vital signs and other key indicators, detailing which physiological functions and indicators PACU caregivers must monitor, and indicating how frequently they must record their observations in the medical record.

Provider collaboration during anesthesia and sedation

<table>
<tr><td><u>R e l e v a n t   s t a n d a r d</u>
TX.1.2</td></tr>
</table>

To satisfy JCAHO standards and, more importantly, to enhance patient safety and quality of care, planning for and management of anesthesia care must be interdisciplinary. It should involve collaboration between all practitioners involved in a specific procedure or in the general oversight of a patient's care. The treatment team should agree on goals and expectations for administration of and recovery from anesthesia or conscious sedation, and team members should involve the patient and the patient's family in this process whenever possible.

Compliance tips

A facility can demonstrate that it provides multidisciplinary anesthesia care—involving nurses, anesthesiologists and/or CRNAs, surgical and medical practitioners, etc.—by reviewing a number of key documents with JCAHO surveyors, including:

- written policies and procedures;
- medical records (especially all anesthesia assessments, anesthesia plans; and progress notes); and
- transfer summaries (see Figure 2.3).

Anesthesia, sedation, and the medication use standards

Relevant standards	
TX.3.3	TX.3.5.6
TX.3.4	TX.3.8
TX.3.5	TX.3.9
TX.3.5.3	

Each year when the JCAHO identifies the standards with which hospitals have the most trouble complying, medication use standards routinely rank among the top ten. In 1998, for instance, the standard that addresses security and control of medication ranked as the second most common source of Type I recommendations. Anesthetics, sedatives, and analgesics are, of course, medications—which means that they're subject to the JCAHO's medication use standards in addition to the anesthesia standards.

Figure 2.3

Transfer summary form

Transfer Summary

Patient name (last, first, middle) _____

Attending physician _____

Principle diagnosis _____

Secondary diagnosis _____

Date of transfer _____ Record # _____

Transfer vital signs
Pulse _____ Oxygen sat _____ BP _____ Temp _____

Allergies _____

Medications _____
_____

Reason for transfer
❏ Observation for apnea
❏ Other   Explain _____
_____

Transfer nursing assessment
_____
_____

Instructions given to patient's primary caregiver
_____
_____

Signature of nurse   Date

Adapted from a form provided by Turville Bay MRI Center. Concept used with permission.

Enactment and enforcement of a medication use policy that addresses a number of key issues (see Exhibit 2) is key to compliance. As with the anesthesia standards, the JCAHO's medication use standards are designed to promote patient safety and quality of care. Organizations that design policies and procedures and train physicians and staff with safety and quality in mind are likely to find that they comply with many of the medication use standards.

What follows is a discussion of the medication use standards that are most relevant to anesthesia care. It addresses the main goals of the medication use standards—controlling access to medications, maintaining the safety and effectiveness of drug treatment, and monitoring outcomes of drug treatment—by focusing on what the JCAHO sees as the five core processes of medication use systems: 1) selection, procurement, and storage; 2) prescribing and ordering; 3) preparation and dispensing; 4) administration; and 5) monitoring effects on the patient (*CAMH*, August 1997 update, TX-20).

Selection, procurement, and storage of medications

The standards that address selection, procurement, and storage of medications call for the creation of a formulary—an inventory of drugs that an organization stocks and allows practitioners to prescribe. The JCAHO expects the development and maintenance of this formulary to be an ongoing, collaborative, and multidisciplinary process that takes into account the needs of an organization's patient population as well as a drug's safety, effectiveness, and cost. However, the JCAHO recognizes that cases may arise in which a patient needs medication not on the formulary, and it expects organizations to establish effective policies and procedures for addressing these cases.

Exhibit 2

Key elements of a medication use policy

A facility must develop and enforce a policy governing medication use. The policy must be consistent with state and federal law and should describe who is authorized to prescribe and/or administer medications. It should also address:

- restrictions on the use of medications under specific conditions or in specific treatment settings;
- requirements for storing and accessing medications when the pharmacy is open and, if relevant, after it has closed for the day;
- procedures for ordering medications;
- guidelines for preparing and administering medications;
- systems for verifying the "five Rs" (right patient, right drug, right dose right time, and right route of administration) prior to administration;
- requirements for monitoring patients after drug administration;
- procedures for identifying and preventing medication allergies and food-drug or drug-drug interactions;
- procedures, consistent with state and federal law, for storing, distributing, and administering controlled substances;
- requirements for obtaining and documenting the informed consent of patients before administration of investigational drugs;
- development of and compliance with the organization's drug formulary;
- procedures for ordering medications not on the formulary;
- requirements for use of vasoactive drugs (e.g., administration by infusion pump may need to be accompanied by carefully documented invasive blood pressure monitoring); and
- procedures for identifying and reporting adverse drug reactions, medication errors, and other adverse drug events.

JCAHO surveyors also expect to see evidence that caregivers are familiar with safe and effective methods for storing medications, and that an organization takes steps to ensure that drugs are stored properly and securely. The standards do not assign one department responsibility for coordinating medication storage and control, but they imply that the pharmacy is probably best prepared to accept it.

Compliance tips

To comply with the standards related to selection, procurement, and storage of medications, an organization should be prepared to show JCAHO surveyors a written copy of its formulary, along with documentation (e.g., meeting minutes) demonstrating that a multidisciplinary task force—with representatives from the medical, pharmacy, nursing, and administrative staffs—reviews the formulary and considers changes to it. In most hospitals, the pharmacy and therapeutics committee performs these reviews and submits formulary recommendations to the medical executive committee for consideration. An organization should have written policies that govern: 1) maintenance of the formulary; 2) procedures for ordering and procuring non-formulary medications; and 3) storage and control of medications. Clinical staff on the formulary-review task force and in patient-care areas should be familiar with these policies.

Prescribing and ordering

The JCAHO requires organizations to institute formal procedures for limiting risks associated with prescribing and ordering medication. The standards identify ten specific areas that organizations need to address, seven of which are relevant to anesthesia and conscious sedation:

1. distribution, administration and/or disposal of controlled medications (such as narcotics and sedatives or hypnotics),

including adequate documentation and record keeping, as required by state and federal law;

2. proper storage, distribution, and control of investigational medications and those in clinical trial;

3. situations in which all or some of a patient's medication orders must be permanently or temporarily canceled, and mechanisms for reinstating them;

4. "as needed" (PRN) prescriptions or orders and times of dose administration;

5. control of sample drugs;

6. distribution of medications to patients at discharge; and

7. procurement, storage, control, and distribution of prepackaged medications obtained from outside sources (*CAMH*, August 1997 update, TX-21).

Compliance tips

Organizations need to have policies and procedures for each of the areas listed above. Among other things, they need to be certain that these policies identify who can prescribe and order medications for patients (by law, this is limited to licensed physicians and, in some states, nurse practitioners and physician assistants) and outline guidelines and procedures regarding the maintenance, availability, and use of patient medication profiles (see Exhibit 3).

Since many anesthetics, sedatives, and analgesics are controlled substances, it's worth highlighting requirements regarding the handling and disposal of controlled substances. State and federal laws addressing this topic are strict. For instance, if a patient does not receive the full contents of a container holding a controlled substance, a licensed

Exhibit 3

The patient medication profile

The patient medication profile (PMP) contains the specific information on a patient's condition, medical history, and medication treatment regimen that caregivers need to ensure the safety of that patient during drug treatment. Every patient who takes medication must have a PMP, and the PMP should be available to and easily accessed by pharmacy staff, nurses, and physicians. All staff involved in patient care should be able to add notations to the PMP, but only a pharmacist should have the authority and ability to change information in a PMP. Ideally, organizations make the PMP available by computer, which facilitates access and may allow more than one person to refer to a patient's profile simultaneously.

Following is a list of information that should generally appear in the PMP:

- the patient's name, birthdate, and gender;
- the patient's current height and weight;
- the patient's problems, symptoms, and/or diagnoses;
- all current medications a patient is taking—including investigational drugs;
- all known allergies and medication sensitivities;
- potential food-drug and/or drug-drug interactions;
- information, if relevant, on a patient's use of illegal drugs;
- information, if relevant, on a patient's misuse of prescription drugs;
- creatinine and BUN values for patients who are over 65 or candidates for kidney dysfunction; and
- body-surface area for chemotherapy patients;

As with all patient information, organizations should take steps to protect the confidentiality of medication profiles.

caregiver must witness the disposal of the leftover portion. In addition, the facility must document: the disposal procedures, the name of the person handling the disposal, and the name of the witness. Most facilities develop adequate policies and procedures for handling controlled substances, but many receive Type I recommendations for failing to comply consistently and/or in all treatment settings with those policies and procedures.

Preparation and dispensing

These standards apply most directly to pharmacy practices. JCAHO expects organizations to comply with all laws, regulations, and practice standards governing the preparation and dispensing of medications and the licensing of individuals who prepare and dispense drugs. Surveyors will also want to see evidence that organizations:

- employ standardized dosing, distribution, and labeling procedures to help prevent medication errors;
- have procedures for preventing patients from receiving expired medications; and
- have pharmacists review all prescriptions and medication orders—except in specific clinical and emergency situations, as outlined in the standards manual (*CAMH*, August 1997 update, TX-21).

The JCAHO insists that diagnoses, known allergies, and other patient information be available to support reviews of prescriptions and orders and help individuals involved in preparing and dispensing medication to:

- facilitate continuity of care;
- create an accurate medication history;

- supplement monitoring of [adverse drug events]; and
- provide safe administration of medications (*CAMH*, August 1997 update, TX-22).

Finally, the JCAHO expects organizations to have effective procedures in place for tracking dispensed medications—including samples—in case of a discontinuation or recall.

Compliance tips

To comply with standards governing preparation and dispensing of drugs, the JCAHO recommends that, among other things, hospitals employ a unit-dose drug distribution system. Most organizations do so, but they also should have written policies and procedures to support and facilitate that system, and to:

- define who has the authority to prepare and dispense medication;
- outline standardized procedures for labeling medication in all preparation areas, including satellite pharmacies;
- mandate that a pharmacist review and initial orders and prescriptions (the policy should also define the scope of these reviews);
- describe the information that must be noted in a patient's chart and medication profile in order to facilitate pharmacist reviews; and
- explain procedures for inspecting drug stocks to ensure patients do not receive expired, recalled, or discontinued medications.

Hospitals should keep copies of relevant policies, laws, and regulations in the pharmacy and in other areas where medication is prepared and dispensed. They should address this information and accepted standards of practice during training and inservice sessions for staff who are authorized to prepare and dispense medications, and they should document the information covered and attendance at these sessions.

Organizations should periodically inspect a sampling of medication orders and patient charts to confirm that staff are complying with relevant policies, and to ensure that orders are supported by appropriate chart documentation. Those inspections should be documented in writing, and inspection reports should be presented as evidence of compliance during a JCAHO survey.

Administration

The standards that apply to medication administration primarily affect the nursing and medical staffs. They are designed to ensure that properly trained and licensed individuals administer medications to patients, that those people verify orders and patient identification before administering drugs, and that they take other steps to augment the safety and effectiveness of drug treatment. In addition to general medication use, these standards address procedures and policies for dealing with investigational medications and medications that patients bring with them to a hospital.

Compliance tips

These standards address what are sometimes called the "five rights" of medication use: right patient, right drug, right dose, right time, and right route of administration. Organizations should have written policies mandating verification of this information and requiring staff to document verification. They should also design and document training and inservice sessions to support these policies. Hospitals might want to consider employing bar coding and other technologies to support and improve the accuracy of verification and identification activities.

Beyond verification activities, these standards require hospitals to design "alternative medication administration systems" for medications that patients bring with them to a hospital and/or that they will be administering to themselves. If, upon admission to a hospital, patients are on medication, the organization should have procedures in place for factoring that existing regimen into all decisions regarding additional medication use. A physician must assess all medications that patients bring with them to the facility—to determine whether use of the drugs is medically appropriate. If patients bring controlled substances or prescription medications to the hospital, the hospital must confirm that written orders authorized use of the drugs; organizations should have a written policy requiring this confirmation. If patients will be self-administering medications, the organization should have written policies that outline procedures for ensuring that patients understand how to administer their medications and for supporting safe, effective self-administration.

Pain management is another issue that's worth discussing in the context of administration of medications and surveillance of medication use. Many hospitals have developed pain management programs that seek to enhance the comfort of patients—often by allowing nurses to administer pain medication on an as-needed basis or giving patients the means to self-administer pain medication. Anesthesiologists should coordinate these programs, and, for the sake of patient safety and quality of care, facilities should control and monitor them as intensely as they control and monitor medication use in any other setting or situation. Lack of appropriate policies and procedures governing pain management programs frequently results in Type I recommendations during JCAHO surveys.

Monitoring the effects of medication on patients

The current standard that requires organizations to assess the effects of medication on patients is designed to ensure that monitoring activities are interdisciplinary, interactive, and continuous. They require physicians, pharmacists, and nurses to work together to monitor effects, to rely on information in medical records and patient medication profiles, and to seek input from patients and their families.

Compliance tips

All monitoring activities must be documented in patient medical records, and organizations should have written policies and procedures that address JCAHO requirements governing drug-effects monitoring. In the context of anesthesia care, hospitals should consider drafting a policy on dealing with malignant hyperthermia, a serious adverse reaction to anesthesia that can cause a patient's body temperature to rise to potentially fatal levels.

An organization's policies should mandate collaboration between physicians, nurses, and pharmacists, should create channels that facilitate and guide this collaboration, and should require caregivers to seek patient input. Among other things, hospital policies and procedures should provide the means for:

- pharmacists to question medication orders that seem inconsistent with aspects of patient diagnoses and/or medication profiles;

- nurses to question abnormal doses or pharmacy deliveries that seem inconsistent with medication orders; and
- nurses, physicians, or pharmacists to report the effects of drug treatment, including unexpected outcomes and adverse drug events.

Educating patients and families about anesthesia and sedation

Relevant standards	
PF.1 & PF.1.1	PF.1.8
PF.1.3	PF.3
PF.1.5	PF.4.1 & PF.4.2

Patient involvement and cooperation are widely viewed as critical to effective medical treatment. For that reason, the JCAHO has long viewed patient and family education as a cornerstone responsibility of hospitals and caregivers. Informed patients, guardians, and surrogate decision-makers are likely to be more compliant with the treatment plan proposed by caregivers. In addition, they may feel less anxious about high-risk procedures like anesthesia and conscious sedation. Effective methods for educating patients and families about anesthesia and sedation—methods that are tailored to each patient's needs and limitations—play an important role in successful anesthesia outcomes.

Educating patients, family members, and/or surrogate decision-makers about anesthesia or sedation means explaining:

- the benefits and desired outcome;
- the likelihood that the procedure involving anesthesia or sedation will be successful;

- the risks and possible complications
- alternative approaches to treatment; and
- the likely effect of postponing or canceling the procedures that call for anesthesia or sedation.

Effective education involves finding ways to overcome language barriers and physical or mental disabilities.

Compliance tips
Organizations should have a policy that outlines procedures and requirements for educating patients and families. They also must ensure that caregivers document the education they provide.

It's important for caregivers to determine how prepared or able individuals are to process information about anesthesia care, and to identify the best methods for educating them. To this end, facilities should consider developing assessment forms that will help caregivers identify the educational needs and limitations of patients, family members, and surrogate decision-makers, including:

- cultural and/or religious preferences;
- literacy and education levels;
- native language(s);
- relevant disabilities (e.g., deafness, dementia, etc.),
- emotional state.

Be sure these forms have enough space to note unique desires, needs, or limitations not covered in enough detail elsewhere (see Figures 2.4a and 2.4b). And make sure your facility provides caregivers with the necessary educational resources by offering them access to translators, video tapes, audio tapes, written materials (see Appendix C), and other materials that will help them respond to the needs of patients, families, and other decision-makers.

Possible food-drug and drug-drug interactions should be a key element of your educational curriculum for anesthesia care. Patients need to understand the risks of such interactions and take steps to help prevent them (e.g., not eating for several hours before a procedure involving anesthesia, telling a practitioner if they have eaten too recently, accurately identifying medications taken before a procedure, etc.). Effective education and communication can help practitioners identify the potential for dangerous interactions, allowing them to modify the anesthesia plan or delay anesthesia until it can be administered safely.

In addition to assessment forms, facilities should consider developing a preoperative program that's designed to teach patients and families basic information about anesthesia. The program might include a brief presentation, during which caregivers:

- explain what will happen before, during, and after anesthesia discuss; and
- use educational tools (handouts, audio tapes, videos, etc.) to describe the qualifications and roles of caregivers involved in the administration of anesthesia and sedation.

Figure 2.4a

Initial knowledge-assessment form

Information Source: ❑ Self   ❑ Spouse   ❑ Parent   ❑ Other:_____

Pre-hospital Teaching: Did you participate in any pre-hospital education?
❑ No   ❑ Yes, describe:_____
_____

Religious/Cultural Practices: Do you have any beliefs or values that we should consider in providing care or education?
❑ No   ❑ Yes, describe:_____
_____

Language(s) spoken: ❑ English   ❑ Other, specify:_____

Educational background: ❑ Grade School   ❑ High School   ❑ Technical
                              ❑ College   ❑ Other, specify:_____

How does patient learn best?   ❑ Seeing   ❑ Hearing   ❑ Doing

Is patient's hearing, sight, or speech impaired?
❑ No   ❑ Yes, describe:_____

Learning aids needed: ❑ Signer   ❑ Interpreter   ❑ None
                        ❑ Other, describe:_____

Motivation: Is patient/family highly motivated to learn?
❑ Yes   ❑ No, describe:_____

Does patient have emotional/family/home concerns that need to be addressed during hospitalization?
❑ No   ❑ Yes, describe:_____

Initial knowledge-assessment form (continued)

Physical Limitations: Do you have any physical limitations that may alter care or limit your learning ability?

❏ No ❏ Yes, describe: _____

Financial Implications: Are there any financial issues or concerns?

❏ No ❏ Yes, describe: _____

Educational Needs: Do you or your family need information on the following?

❏ Current illness	❏ Medications	❏ Community
❏ Homecare	❏ Equipment	❏ Access to follow-up care
❏ Rehab techniques	❏ Diet/nutrition	❏ None
❏ Personal hygiene	❏ Restraints	❏ Other: _____

Is access to schooling needed? (For school-age and adolescent patients with long periods of hospitalization)

❏ No ❏ Yes

Did you receive a copy of the Patient Rights Booklet?

❏ Yes ❏ No, explain _____

Do you or your family have any questions?

❏ No ❏ Yes, explain _____

Educational needs by priority (as appropriate)

1._____
2._____
3._____

_____
Signature   Time   Date

_____
Signature   Time   Date

Source: Joan Iacono, RN, MSN, MBA and Ann Campbell, RN, MSN, Patient and Family Education: The Compliance Guide to the JCAHO Standards *(Marblehead, MA: Opus Communications, 1997), p. 12.*

Figure 2.4b

Educational needs and abilities assessment

Speech: ❏ Normal ❏ Problems: _____

Language(s) spoken: ❏ English ❏ Other(s): _____

Memory problems: ❏ No ❏ Yes:

        Recent: ❏ No ❏ Yes: _____

        Remote: ❏ No ❏ Yes

Learning problems: ❏ No ❏ Yes: _____

Learning style: ❏ Visual ❏ Auditory ❏ Touch

Education level: (check the highest level)
❏ Grade school ❏ High School
❏ College ❏ Postgraduate

Patient's perception of reading skills: ❏ Excellent ❏ Good ❏ Poor

What does patient know about his/her health problem(s)? _____
_____

Cultural/spiritual: Are there religious, traditional, ethnic, or cultural practices that need to be addressed during care?
❏ No ❏ Yes: _____

Is there any way the hospital can assist patient's with your religious practices?
❏ No ❏ Yes: _____

Pre-hospital teaching: Did patient participate in pre-hospital education?
❏ No ❏ Yes: _____

How best do you learn new information?
❏ Reading ❏ Audiotapes ❏ Return demonstration
❏ Video ❏ Listening ❏ Touching

Caregiver assessment: Is patient/family motivated to learn?
❏ Yes ❏ No: _____

Educational needs and abilities assessment (continued)

Is patient/family ready to learn?
❏ Yes ❏ No: _____

_____

Is patient beginning to ask questions about his/her conditon or treatment?
❏ No ❏ Yes: _____

_____

Barriers to learning: Is the patient emotionally impaired in any way?
❏No ❏ Yes: _____

_____

Is the patient physically impaired in any way?
❏ No ❏ Yes: _____

_____

Does the patient have learning disabilities or other cognitive impairments?
❏ No ❏ Yes: _____

_____

Source: Joan, Iacono, RN, MSN, MBA and Ann Campbell, RN, MSN, Patient and Family Education: The Compliance Guide to the JCAHO Standards *(Marblehead, MA: Opus Communications, 1997, p. 13.*

Anesthesia, sedation, and continuity of care

R e l e v a n t s t a n d a r d s	
CC.4	CC.6 & CC.6.1
CC.5	CC.7

It is not unusual for several caregivers to treat a patient over the course of one or more treatment episodes. For that treatment to be as safe and effective as possible, the transfer of patient information between caregivers, treatment settings, and treatment episodes must be efficient and flawless. The JCAHO's continuity of care (CC) standards require seamless transitions across treatment settings and between caregivers.

In the context of anesthesia care, continuity is dependent on three factors: 1) patient and family education, 2) information management, and 3) practitioner collaboration and communication. If patients, family members, and surrogate decision-makers are not educated effectively about anesthesia care, they may not provide the information necessary to ensure continuity of care across settings and between caregivers. Likewise, failure to note that information and other key facts about the patient in the medical record (i.e., diagnosis, treatment plan, known allergies, etc.) may compromise the quality of anesthesia care and the safety of the patient.

Compliance tips
Facilities must develop clear policies and standardized systems and protocols that require and encourage effective collaboration, communication, and information management. These policies must include a plan for patient care services that requires staff who steer patients through the continuum of care to:

- assess patient needs upon admission;
- follow predetermined criteria for admission to all care settings (including, of course, those associated with anesthesia care);
- explain to patients and their families the costs of and alternatives to the planned course of treatment;
- ensure that discharges, transfers, and referrals do not disrupt treatment regimens;

- document in the medical record caregiver rationale for discharging, transferring, or referring a patient; and
- follow procedures to ensure patient information is available to caregivers when they need it.

Facilities should constantly train and retrain caregivers to ensure they are familiar with the policies and operate consistently and effectively within those systems. Whenever possible they should develop forms and checklists that reduce the chances that crucial patient information gets overlooked or miscommunicated. Humans make mistakes, and the more organizations can provide tools to support, prompt, and remind caregivers, the better off patients are likely to be. As with many other JCAHO standards, documentation of the steps taken to ensure compliance is a key part of demonstrating compliance. Organizations should be prepared to show surveyors written copies of their policies, procedures, and protocols. They should also take minutes and keep attendance lists at all training sessions so they can document their efforts and caregiver participation.

Anesthesia, sedation, and performance improvement

Relevant standards	
PI.3–PI.5	IM.8
MS.8–MS.8.1.6	LD.1.4
MS.8.3 & MS.8.4	LD.4.2–LD.4.3.2

New JCAHO standards outlining requirements for data-driven performance improvement took effect in 1999. They are designed to be less prescriptive than past requirements, emphasizing the importance of designing and maintaining a quality monitoring and improvement program that is tailored to the specific needs of an organization's patient population. They include fewer required performance measures and now identify suggested indicators that organizations can elect to monitor if there's a reason or need to do so. The remaining required measures target "high-risk, high-volume, problem-prone areas," including a number that relate to anesthesia and conscious sedation:

- medication use;
- operative and other invasive and noninvasive procedures that can place patients at risk (e.g., CAT scans and MRIs);
- use of blood and blood products (*CAMH*, August 1998 update, PI-11).

Hospitals must assign, in writing, responsibility for implementing the improvement initiatives that result from PI analysis.

When relevant, performance-related information and findings must be forwarded to hospital leadership. The JCAHO expects hospital leaders to:

- understand performance improvement (PI) techniques;
- adopt a specific approach to PI;
- require and encourage implementation of that approach as part of an effective PI program;
- allocate resources needed for effective PI; and
- participate in PI activities.

The JCAHO expects members of the medical staff to participate in PI analysis of all processes that are dependent upon licensed independent practitioners. The standards mention four specific processes, each of which relate to anesthesia or conscious sedation:

- medical assessment and treatment of patients;
- use of medications;
- use of blood and blood components; and
- use of operative and other procedures (*CAMH,* February 1999 update, MS-13).

ORYX

Over the past two years, the JCAHO has been shaping what it calls the ORYX initiative, which is designed to

- allow the JCAHO to track hospital performance on an ongoing basis;
- encourage an ongoing, data-driven approach to performance improvement; and
- establish standardized "core measures" that allows the JCAHO to compare a hospital's performance against national norms.

As this book went to press, the JCAHO announced five core measures that hospitals must begin to track and report in 2000:

- acute myocardial infarction;
- congestive heart failure;
- pneumonia;
- pregnancy-related conditions; and
- surgical procedures and complications.

In addition, the JCAHO expects organizations to choose and report quarterly performance data for six additional measures that affect 30 percent of their patient population.

Sentinel events

The current standards require organizations to analyze "undesirable patterns or trends in performance and sentinel events" (see Exhibit 4) and implement "changes that will lead to improved performance." The JCAHO identifies several types of incident that organizations must analyze, including three that relate to anesthesia and conscious sedation:

- significant adverse events associated with anesthesia care;
- significant adverse drug reactions; and
- significant medication errors (*CAMH*, August 1998 update, PI-16–PI-17).

Compliance tips

Performance improvement must be a priority for all healthcare organizations, something they use proactively to fulfill their missions and to ensure the quality of care they provide. During interview sessions, surveyors will gauge how well physicians and hospital staff understand your organization's approach to PI (e.g., the FOCUS-PDCA method, the FADE method, etc.). They'll want to see evidence that your PI program receives support and oversight at the highest levels. They'll also want assurances that people at all levels of the organization and medical staff understand their PI roles and responsibilities and participate in improvement projects.

During interviews with caregivers, quality staff, leaders, and others, JCAHO surveyors may ask for examples of anesthesia-related incidents

Exhibit 4

Sentinel events

In 1998 and 1999, the JCAHO enacted a policy and standards that target unexpected incidents "involving death or serious physical or psychological injury, or the risk thereof" (CAMH, August 1998 update, AC-5). The JCAHO refers to such incidents as sentinel events and identifies five specific categories of event that warrant immediate action:

1. a patient suicide in a setting where the patient receives care around the clock
2. an infant abduction or discharge to the wrong family
3. a rape
4. a hemolytic reaction involving administration of blood or blood products having major blood group incompatibilities; or
5. surgery on the wrong patient or wrong body part

The stated goal of the policy and standards is to identify, investigate, and attempt to eliminate flaws in treatment systems and processes that put patients at risk. Any time patients die unexpectedly or experience a major, permanent loss of function that's not related to the natural course of their illnesses or conditions, organizations are encouraged to report the incident to the Joint Commission within five business days.[1] In addition, the JCAHO requires organizations to analyze such events

---

[1] Reporting of sentinel events is currently voluntary. However, at the time this book was written, most experts advised organizations not to report sentinel events to the JCAHO for liability reasons. Because the Joint Commission does not have peer review status, it is possible that plaintiffs' attorneys could compel the JCAHO to reveal the information contained in verbal or written sentinel event reports. However, there is almost unanimous agreement that, whether they report them or not, it's important for healthcare organizations to respond to sentinel and other adverse events by investigating their root causes and redesigning systems and processes in an effort to prevent similar events from occurring.

Sentinel events *(continued)*

no later than 45 days after learning of them. Once that analysis is complete, organizations must take measurable steps designed to prevent similar incidents.

Organizations that do not complete sentinel event investigations within 45 days will be placed on accreditation watch, a designation that publicly indicates they experienced a sentinel event and have not cooperated with the JCAHO to reconcile it. If the organization does not complete an investigation within two weeks of going on accreditation watch, its accreditation will be revoked.

JCAHO surveyors are likely to ask for your definition of a sentinel event. They'll also want to discuss your methods for identifying and investigating them, and for designing systems improvements following those investigations. They are likely to ask organizations if they've experienced any sentinel events since their last survey and, since it's widely believed that all hospitals experience several per year, they'll react skeptically to organizations that claim they have not had any. Hosptial leaders are responsible for ensuring that an organization establishes and implements systems for identifying and managing sentinel events.

that your organization would consider adverse. They're also likely to ask about the performance indicators and monitoring mechanisms your organization uses to identify such incidents (and related incidents, such as adverse drug reactions, medication errors, or unexpected admissions following outpatient surgery). They may also ask relevant personnel to discuss a recent anesthesia-related PI project undertaken within your organization. Make sure, therefore, that relevant members of the medical and hospital staffs are familiar with your policies and procedures for monitoring the quality of anesthesia care, and formalize those and other PI policies and procedures by drafting a system-wide performance improvement plan. Your plan must address JCAHO requirements regarding monitoring and improvement of anesthesia care and other processes. In general, it should:

- outline the performance indicators for anesthesia care (see Figure 2.5) and other clinical and nonclinical processes that your organization monitors;
- describe how your organization identifies and capitalizes on opportunities to improve anesthesia care and other clinical or nonclinical processes; and
- demonstrate your organization's commitment to PI as an ongoing, collaborative, and multidisciplinary process.

Effective PI programs are data-driven and produce measurable improvement initiatives, so JCAHO surveyors will also expect your plan to:

- outline effective mechanisms for capturing information about quality of care (e.g., voluntary reporting by caregivers and/or regular auditing of medical records and performance-related databases);

- mandate the use of formal tools and techniques for evaluating performance data;
- require members of your PI taskforces to design and implement measurable improvement initiatives based on the data they've collected and analyzed; and
- require members of your PI taskforces to track the results of improvement initiatives and revise them, as needed.

An organization's PI plan is usually the primary source of documented evidence regarding compliance. However, other documents that will

Figure 2.5

Anesthesia indicators

1. CNS complication within 2 post procedure days.
2. Peripheral neurologic deficit within 2 post procedure days.
3. Acute MI within 2 post procedure days.
4. Cardiac arrest within 2 post procedure days.
5. Respiratory arrest within 2 post procedure days.
6. Death within 2 post procedure days.
7. Unplanned admission within 1 post procedure day of outpatient surgery.
8. Unplanned admission to an ICU within 1 post procedure day of surgery.
9. Pulmonary edema within 1 post procedure day.
10. Aspiration pneumonitis within 2 post procedure days.
11. Postural headache within 4 post procedure days of a spinal or epidural anesthetic.
12. Dental injury during anesthetic care.
13. Ocular injury during anesthetic care.

Source: St. Joseph's Hospital and Medical Center, Phoenix, Arizona.

help to demonstrate compliance include an organization's mission or vision statement, minutes and attendance lists from PI task force meetings, and reports documenting the goals and results of improvement initiatives.

Anesthesia, sedation, and leadership

Relevant standards	
LD.1.3.3 & LD.1.3.3.1	LD.3
LD.1.6	LD.3.2
LD.1.7 & LD.1.7.1	LD.3.4
LD.2	

JCAHO leadership (LD) standards are relevant to this discussion of anesthesia and sedation because the Joint Commission expects hospital and medical staff leaders to:

- decide which clinical services (including anesthesia and sedation) are consistent with the organization's and/or Medical Executive Committee's (MEC's) mission (see Figure 2.6) and should be available to patients;
- coordinate provision of those services within and across departments; and
- oversee and improve the quality of those services.

The JCAHO holds leaders responsible for ensuring that patients receive a comparable level of care in all treatment settings and from all practitioners within an organization. This requirement is particularly relevant to anesthesia because practitioners perform procedures involving anesthesia in a wide range of settings. It has become a more complcated leadership requirement as the development of integrated health systems has expanded the range of settings within organizations where patients receive anesthesia, sedation, and other services.

As is the case in all clinical departments, the leadership of the anesthesia department must prepare a written document outlining its goals and scope of services. The JCAHO expects the department's goals to be consistent with the organization's overall mission, and the scope of available anesthesia services must adequately address the needs of the organization's patient population. Department leaders must provide support services and staffing that are consistent with the scope of services outlined.

Figure 2.6	Sample MEC mission statement

The mission of the Executive Committee of the medical staff of St. Joseph's Hospital and Medical Center is

- to provide proactive leadership for the organized medical staff in this rapidly changing healthcare environment.
- to ensure the provision of quality patient care and to measure the value of services rendered.
- to assure that physicians are appropriately credentialed for membership and privileged commensurate with their individual training and experience.
- to provide a forum to discuss and mediate other physician issues.
- to recommend action to the Board of Directors of Mercy Healthcare Arizona regarding items of concern to the Medical Staff.
- to assist in the strategic planning and direction taken by Mercy Healthcare Arizona and Catholic Healthcare West.

Source: St. Joseph's Hospital and Medical Center, Phoenix, AZ

Compliance tips

Organizations and anesthesia departments should be prepared to discuss their mission and scope of services with JCAHO surveyors. They must also develop policy and procedure documents that are consistent with the requirements outlined above, and they should document steps taken by hospital and medical staff leaders to ensure compliance with those policies and procedures.

In general, an organization's anesthesia policy should address the following leadership and management issues:

- the role of anesthesia services within the organization's overall goals, mission, and scope of services;
- credentialing and privileging requirements for anesthesia practitioners (see Chapter 3);
- system-wide protocols governing anesthesia care;
- guidelines for ensuring a comparable level of anesthesia care throughout the organization;
- expectations regarding collaboration between providers, departments, and specialties; and
- performance indicators and improvement requirements for anesthesia services.

Anesthesia, sedation, and the environment of care

Relevant standards	
EC.1.3	EC.2.2
EC.1.5–EC.1.9	EC.2.4–EC.2.9
EC.2.1	EC.2.11–EC.2.14

While there is some unavoidable risk associated with anesthesia and sedation, facilities must take steps to minimize it. Patients receiving anesthesia and sedation often lose consciousness, may be fully or partially immobilized, and may lose their protective reflexes. In those instances, they're dependent on medical equipment, skilled practitioners, and hospital staff to preserve their health and safety. When patients agree to undergo procedures involving sedation, for example, they trust that their caregivers will know how to react if they lose their protective reflexes and that the equipment needed to keep them alive will be on hand and working reliably. Likewise, patients trust that facilities will have policies, procedures, and equipment in place to deal with fires, natural disasters, and other emergencies that have the potential to compromise their safety.

Compliance tips

To comply with the JCAHO's environment of care standards affecting anesthesia care, facilities must develop and implement management plans that outline key requirements (e.g., maintenance schedules, inspection schedules, testing/drill schedules, staff training, etc.) in a number of areas, including:

- safety;
- emergency preparedness (in case of fire, flood, tornado, riot, etc.);
- life safety;
- medical equipment (e.g., ventilators, etc.); and
- utility systems (e.g., electricity, water, telecommunications systems, etc.)

The requirements and policies outlined in these management plans must conform to state and federal laws, existing healthcare regulations, and current standards.

Organizations must hold training sessions and drills for all shifts to ensure that staff are prepared to respond to fires, equipment failures, power outages, and other emergencies that affect the environment of care and put patients at risk. They must document the occurrence and results of these tests, document staff participation in them, and address flaws in their management plan and/or deficiencies in staff knowledge or performance.

Managing human resources for anesthesia and sedation

Relevant standards	
HR.2	HR.3

Facilities must be able to document that the practitioners and hospital staff involved in anesthesia care have enough training and experience to treat patients safely and effectively in all settings. Staffing in operating rooms, PACUs, and special care units must be consistent with state and federal law, regulatory requirements, and a hospital's internal policies.

Hospital and physician leaders must develop systems to measure, maintain, and improve staff competency. Leaders involved directly in anesthesia care must assess staff competency in operating rooms, PACUs, and special care units. They must plan and implement continuing medical education (CME) programs for the anesthesia department and should consider adopting the ASA's guidelines for CME (see page 145).

Staff training, competence, and experience must suit the needs of an organization's patient population, and caregiver competence must extend to all patients regardless of age or illness. In addition, all staff should be able to demonstrate that, for both high-risk, high-volume and high-risk, low-volume procedures, they can competently treat patients of all ages served by a facility.

Compliance tips
Facilities should develop a policy on human resources that applies to all settings where and times when providers administer anesthesia. The policy should require the following:

- members of the medical and hospital staff have sufficient training and experience to provide anesthesia services for the facility's patient population;
- the facility measures, maintains, and improves the performance of staff involved in anesthesia care; and
- the facility makes CME programs on anesthesia care available to all relevant staff.

The facility should also document actions and activities that indicate compliance with and enforcement of these policies.

Information management and anesthesia care

Relevant standards	
IM.5	IM.7.3.3
IM.7.3	IM.7.4
IM.7.3.1	IM.9

Because anesthesia care is provided in different settings throughout the facility, medical records serve as the key source of information about a patient, and a key vehicle for ensuring the continuity and quality of care. In the context of anesthesia care, for instance, practitioners need information on past hospitalizations, surgeries, and procedures—especially as it pertains to a patient's past experiences with anesthesia or sedation. They also need to know about allergies, current diagnoses, results of relevant lab tests, and many other facts about a patient's condition or status—all of which affect decisions about anesthesia and sedation. Organizations must, in short, have policies and procedures in place for ensuring that information in the medical record is:

- accurate;
- up to date;
- formatted consistently to ensure that caregivers can find what they need and are less likely to overlook key details; and
- available to practitioners and caregivers when they need it.

In ensuring caregiver access to patient information, however, organizations must also take documented steps to keep unauthorized individuals from accessing confidential information about patients.

Organizations must carefully monitor practitioner documentation to ensure that all pertinent information gets charted. For instance, practitioners must document all operative, diagnostic, and therapeutic procedures—including any use of anesthesia or sedation. Caregivers monitoring the patient's recovery from anesthesia or sedation must document the patient's vital signs and mental status. They also must document administration of medications, fluids, blood or blood products. And, they're required to make note of unexpected events or complications, steps taken to resolve the situation, and the effect on the patient.

If a patient is discharged from the facility but requires continuing care, the patient's medical record must contain all information needed to guide that continuing care. Documents in the record should include summaries of diagnoses, procedures, medication use, allergies, and discharge instructions.

In addition to requiring organizations to manage patient information carefully, the JCAHO IM standards also insist that physicians and other caregivers have access to patient-care literature through medical journals, medical reference materials, and other such resources. These resources should include information that helps anesthesiologists, certified registered nurse anesthetists (CRNAs), and other authorized caregivers provide safe, effective anesthesia care.

Compliance tips

To comply with the JCAHO IM standards affecting anesthesia care, organizations must develop and enforce policies and procedures that are consistent with the requirements outlined above. They should periodically audit medical records to ensure the records include documentation for all necessary aspects of preanesthesia care, anesthesia care, and postanesthesia care. Organizations should also consider adopting the guidelines and standards laid out in the ASA's "Documentation of Anesthesia Care" (see page 149).

Infection control in anesthesia settings

Relevant standards
IC.2–IC.5

Due to the risks posed during anesthesia care by blood-borne infectious agents—such as hepatitis, HIV, and airborne tuberculosis, healthcare facilities must vigilantly seek to prevent the transmission of disease from patient to patient or from patient to caregiver. A facility must dedicate educational resources to reducing the risks of transmission of infectious agents. It must also have policies for responding to and treating incidents that pose a significant threat of infection—like needle sticks and contact in other ways with potentially contaminated blood and other substances.

An organization's infection control policies must apply to all settings where anesthesia is administered. It should outline conditions of employment that are designed to reduce the risk of infection, such as mandatory tuberculosis screenings. Hospital and medical staff at risk of exposure to blood or bodily fluids should be encouraged to receive a hepatitis B vaccine, and personnel with active respiratory or cutaneous infections should not have direct contact with patients. The organization should also hold, and require employee participation in, periodic training sessions on infection control.

Compliance tips
Facilities must have written policies and procedures in place that address infection control and are consistent with guidelines developed by agencies such as the Centers for Disease Control and Prevention. Policies must conform with state and federal laws and regulations, and they should address the following issues:

- sterilization;
- disinfection;
- barrier precautions;
- handling sterile supplies;

- sanitation for rooms and supplies;
- hand washing;
- appropriate clothing, including eyewear and masks;
- handling and disposal of needles and other sharp objects; and
- adherence to standard infection control precautions.

Facilities must also document activities related to compliance with JCAHO IC standards, including enforcement actions and relevant training sessions.

Medical staff standards and anesthesia care

Relevant standards	
MS.1–MS.1.1.3	MS.5.14–MS.5.15.7
MS.2.3	MS.6.2–MS.6.2.2.1
MS.2.3.2–MS.2.3.6	MS.6.4–MS.6.5.2
MS.2.5	MS.6.8–MS.7.2.1
MS.4–MS.4.2.1.15	

Anesthesiologists are members of a medical staff, the governing body for the licensed independent practitioners allowed to practice medicine in an organization. The JCAHO no longer requires organizations to have a single, organized medical staff, recognizing that managed care and the development of far-flung health systems makes that an unwieldy structure in many cases. However, the JCAHO still requires LIPs to practice within a governing structure, and it prohibits individual facilities from maintaining more than one medical staff.

The medical staff is responsible for the quality of services provided by its members and accountable to an organization's board (or other governing body). Medical staff members must have delineated clinical privileges (see below and Chapter 3) identifying the services and procedures they're authorized to order and perform (e.g., administration of anesthesia and/or sedation), and they are subject to the medical staff's bylaws, policies, rules, and regulations. Like all physician leaders, anesthesiologists must play an active role in medical staff leadership, quality monitoring, and performance improvement.

If an anesthesia department or group participates in graduate medical education programs, the organization's rules and regulations must outline requirements for medical staff supervision of interns, residents, and fellows. Medical staff members who serve as supervisors usually must countersign medical record entries written by house staff.

If certified registered nurse anesthetists (CRNAs) practice in an organization—whether they are employed by the hospital, by other practitioners, or are self-employed—they must practice in accordance with all laws and regulations, some of which vary by state. Some states, for instance, insist that an anesthesiologist supervise or direct all care that CRNAs provide. CRNAs must also comply with the internal policies and procedures of the facilities in which they practice, and, when relevant, with the bylaws, rules, and regulations that govern the facility's medical staff. These medical staff governing documents should include criteria that allow for easy identification of instances when CRNAs must consult with a LIP. For instance, CRNAs may be allowed to perform all or part of a patient's history and physical—including the assessment of anesthesia risks—but medical staff policies and/or state and federal guidelines may require physician confirmation of the findings.

If a facility has an anesthesia department, it must have designated leadership—including a director with board certification or a comparable level of documented experience and skill. The chair or director of the anesthesia department—or of other departments that have need for anesthesia and sedation services (e.g., surgery, radiology, etc.)—is responsible for:

- helping the facility identify the types of services needed to meet the patient population's needs;
- overseeing the clinical activities of the department;
- developing department policies and procedures,
- developing criteria for privileging;
- making recommendations regarding granting of clinical privileges; and
- ensuring the effectiveness of quality monitoring and performance improvement within the department.

Practitioners who are qualified to provide unsupervised patient care must have delineated clinical privileges that clearly describe the patient care services they are allowed to provide, and organizations must have systems in place to ensure that no practitioner orders or provides services and procedures that lie outside the scope of his or her privileges. Decisions to grant privileges should be based upon a review of specific criteria, including the specialty of the provider requesting privileges, the provider's training and experience, age-specific competencies, the risk associated with the procedures and services in question, and the requesting practitioner's ability to manage and address those risks.

Requirements regarding privileges extend to physicians and physician groups with exclusive contracts—a fact that is relevant to this discussion since anesthesiology is one of four service areas often provided on a contract basis (the other areas are radiology, pathology, and emergency medicine). The medical staff must define and approve a system for granting privileges to physicians who provide contracted services, and the medical staff's bylaws, credentials policy, and/or rules and regulations should explain this system.

For complicated or risky procedures, organizations should consider requiring evidence of specialized training and expertise. With regard to anesthesia and sedation, for instance, organizations might want to develop special criteria for practitioners seeking privileges to insert pulmonary artery catheters, provide anesthesia during open heart surgery, perform invasive pain management procedures, or provide anesthesia care for infants.

In organizations that have clinical departments, LIPs must be assigned to departments that provide and monitor the services for which they've been granted privileges. If the organization does not have clinical departments, the medical staff's bylaws must outline formal processes for granting privileges and reviewing the quality of care provided by individual practitioners.

The JCAHO requires practitioners to participate in continuing medical education programs. Facilities must document their participation in these programs, and factor it into decisions regarding renewal of privileges and reappointment to the medical staff.

Compliance tips

Organizations must develop medical staff governing documents (bylaws, policies and procedures, and rules and regulations) that are consistent with all requirements noted above. At bare minimum, the bylaws should:

- outline the formal structure of the medical staff practicing within a facility or facilities;
- create a medical executive committee to oversee medical staff operations;
- outline a fair hearing and appeals process to protect the rights of medical staff members;
- address issues of unacceptable clinical practice, including: disregard for rules, mental or physical impairment, disruptive behavior, and unethical behavior.

Beyond the bylaws, organizations should develop, implement, and enforce the following:

- a credentialing policy or manual;
- a clinical consultation policy;
- other relevant clinical policies (including a conscious sedation policy)
- manuals outlining guidelines, policies and methods for all clinical departments (including anesthesiology); and
- a plan for assessing physician performance and improvement.

All medical staff members must receive a copy of these documents, as well as copies of significant revisions. The requirements and standards outlined in the medical staff governing documents also must be consistent with all relevant laws and regulations, and organizations must be able to document compliance with these documents. Indeed, staff failure to abide by organizational policies is one of the most common reasons organizations receive Type I recommendations during JCAHO surveys.

The JCAHO standards do not require organizations to establish clinical departments. In fact, for small hospitals a non-departmentalized approach can be quite effective. However, in facilities that do have clinical departments, department heads must be board certified or have an equivalent level of skill and experience. Organizations should be prepared to show JCAHO surveyors documented procedures for selecting department heads and a written job description outlining the department head's responsibility. They should also be able to demonstrate that they choose departmental leadership carefully.

Delineated clinical privileges must be individual-specific and based on demonstrated current competence; the JCAHO prohibits granting of blanket privileges to all physicians in a department or on a medical staff. Careful compliance with this requirement can help organizations begin to meet the JCAHO requirements calling for comparable levels of care.

Clinical privileges for contract physicians—a common status for anesthesiologists—are usually granted through normal or routine privileging channels. However, organizations should probably consult their legal counsel when determining what happens to those privileges if the contract is lost.

Finally, organizations must establish mechanisms to ensure that licensed independent practitioners order and perform only those services for which they have privileges, and that non-physician practitioners (e.g., CRNAs) perform only those services outlined in their job descriptions or scope-of-service documents. To this end, organizations often circulate lists of practitioners who are authorized to order or perform risky or uncommon procedures; these lists and other mechanisms are commonly known as "point of patient" checks.

Credentialing and Privileging Requirements

To help protect patient safety and ensure the quality of care patients receive, hospitals and ambulatory care centers are required to assess and verify the credentials of licensed independent practitioners (LIPs) who apply for appointment to that organization's medical staff. Credentialing involves verifying from a primary source that individual practitioners meet the organization's minimum requirements for appointment to the medical staff and have the medical education, training, and experience outlined on their application. Appointment should last for no more than two years, at which point practitioners must apply for reappointment.

Once an organization verifies a practitioner's credentials and approves his or her application for membership on the medical staff, the organization must define the accepted scope of practice for that practitioner. This second process, known commonly as privileging, involves further review of experience and competence to determine whether the practitioner is qualified to perform the clinical procedures he or she has asked to perform (see Figure 3.1).

The permission to perform procedures and provide patient care services that an organization grants practitioners is known as delineated

Figure 3.1		
Privileging guidelines for conscious sedation		
Privilege requested	**Minimum formal training**	**Required previous experience**
Conscious sedation or sedation and analgesia	Successful completion of an accredited three-year residency in anesthesiology or Where appropriate, graduation from a nurse anesthesia educational program accredited by the American Association of Nurse Anesthetists' Council on Certification of Nurse Anesthesia Educational Programs (or the council's predecessor) or Successful completion of a residency (with or without a subspecialty fellowship) wherein the LIP received education, training, and experience to administer and/or supervise conscious sedation (this would apply to physicians other than anesthesiologists, such as pulmonologists, gastroenterologists, surgeons, or cardiologists)	Performance of conscious sedation (also known as sedation and analgesia) for at least 50 patients over the past 12 months

Adapted from: Beverly E. Pybus, CMSC, The Privileging Quick Reference Guide *(Marblehead, MA: Opus Communications, 1998), 33–34.*

clinical privileges. Before considering applications for a specific privilege, a healthcare facility's medical staff leadership and board must:

- approve a plan for the facility to offer the procedure or service in question; and
- define criteria for determining which practitioners are qualified to perform the procedure or service in question.

Healthcare facilities must pay close attention to credentialing and privileging for anesthesia because it is a specialized, high-risk area of practice. The Joint Commission on Accreditation of Healthcare Organizations (JCAHO) recognizes these risks and has developed specific standards to govern anesthesia care in accredited facilities (see Chapter 2). The credentialing and privileging requirements included in these standards will receive additional attention in this chapter—along with a discussion on best practices for credentialing and privileging LIPs who provide anesthesia care.

Credentialing, privileging, and anesthesia

The JCAHO requirements for credentialing and privileging apply, of course, to anesthesia care and the LIPs who provide it: anesthesiologists, surgeons, dentists, certified registered nurse anesthetists (CRNA),[1] etc. They require that a facility's medical staff include only licensed physicians and/or appropriately licensed non-physician practitioners who by law and the medical staff's bylaws are authorized to treat

---

[1] Some credentialing experts say it is not always necessary to grant privileges to CRNAs because in many states and/or healthcare organizations CRNAs are not considered LIPs, which makes them ineligible for medical staff membership. According to these experts, only LIPs—practitioners who by law and medical staff bylaws are allowed to direct and provide patient care without supervision—are required to secure appointment to a medical staff, and only medical staff members are required to have delineated clinical privileges. In states that do not recognize CRNAs as LIPs, or in organizations that make them hospital employees (like RNs) rather having them apply for appointment to the medical staff, it's not necessary to privilege CRNAs. Instead, the facility's human resources department should develop a CRNA job description and draft scope-of-practice documentation (outlining the specific patient-care services an individual CRNA can provide) for each CRNA authorized to practice in the facility.

patients without supervision (state laws and/or organizational bylaws may not allow CRNAs to practice without supervision; see previous page, note 1). All medical staff members—including anesthesiologists—must have delineated privileges and are required to participate in performance improvement initiatives.

Factoring in conscious sedation

The JCAHO does not require organizations to grant specific privileges for the provision of conscious sedation (also known as sedation and analgesia; see Chapter 1, note 1), which involves administration of sedatives, analgesics, or hypnotics in doses or under conditions that can cause patients to lose their protective airway reflexes. However, conscious sedation is risky enough, and JCAHO surveyors ask about it often enough (see page 6), that organizations should consider enacting a conscious sedation policy that requires practitioners to apply for conscious sedation privileges independently of anesthesia privileges. Accredited organizations that don't require specific privileges for conscious sedation should have a conscious sedation policy (see Chapter 1) that only allows practitioners with anesthesia privileges to order and administer (or oversee the administration of) sedation if the sedated patient has a reasonable chance of losing his or her protective reflexes. That's because the JCAHO considers loss of reflexes to be an element of anesthesia care and applies its anesthesia standards to instances in which sedation prompts loss of reflexes.

The American Society of Anesthesiologists' "Guidelines for Delineation of Clinical Privileges in Anesthesiology" (see page 167) can serve as a valuable resource for organizations as they develop criteria upon which to judge requests for anesthesiology privileges. Many of those guidelines are consistent with the JCAHO requirements. Ultimately, however, organizations must evaluate requests for privileges by answering a series of key questions, including:

- Do our bylaws allow practitioners to perform the requested procedure(s)?
- Does the requesting practitioner have a current license to practice medication?
- Do federal or state laws bar the practitioner from providing the requested service(s)?
- Is the practitioner's training or documented clinical experience consistent with his or her request for privileges?
- Does the practitioner's peer-review history and outcomes data indicate current competence?
- Is the practitioner mentally and physically able to provide the requested services?
- Do the practitioner's references and recommendations check out?

Is board certification required?

The JCAHO's medical staff standards require board certification or a comparable level of competence for department directors who are elected or appointed after January 1, 1992. In general, however, the JCAHO does not require anesthesiologists and other physicians seeking medical staff membership or delineated clinical privileges to be board certified. Nonetheless, many organizations view board certification as a strong indicator of skill and competence; they may choose to require board certification in the clinical specialty area(s) for which the privileges are granted—either for all practitioners applying or for less experienced practitioners (e.g., those who completed residencies after a certain date). Regardless of whether they choose to require board certification, organizations must apply their requirements uniformly to all practitioners.

Tailored privileges

Because some facilities provide anesthesia care that is complex or extensive, physicians at those facilities often must demonstrate competency in specialized areas. This may include:

- high-risk or premature neonates;
- patients who are in critical condition or intensive care;
- patients experiencing acute or chronic pain;
- patients undergoing open-heart or transplant surgery;
- patients undergoing high-risk obstetrical procedures;
- patients undergoing other high-risk, specialized procedures for which practitioners need additional education, training, and experience.

In these circumstances, procedure-specific privileges are tailored for physicians with general privileges and the skills required for such highly specialized or technologically advanced care.

Credentialing for ambulatory centers

Credentialing and privileging requirements have been problematic for ambulatory centers—where more and more procedures involving anesthesia and sedation are performed, and where the range of settings and practitioners providing care may make it harder for organizations to ensure that patients receive a comparable level of care. The JCAHO can survey ambulatory facilities that are affiliated with hospitals under either its hospital or its ambulatory standards. In either case, the JCAHO standards for credentialing a practitioner are consistent:

- The center must have a defined process of credentialing, privileging, and appointment, with reappointment taking place at least every two years.
- Anesthesia practitioners must provide evidence of, and the facility must perform primary-source verification of, all relevant credentials, including licensure, education, training, and experience.

Free-standing centers have been known to accept at face value the verification activities of a hospital or to assume that membership on a hospital medical staff guarantees adequate credentials verification. Neither approach is acceptable. All organizations need to gather primary-source verification of practitioner credentials before granting appointments. They should do so with equal care and rigor, following four basic rules:

1. *Credential all practitioners*. The center's credentialing requirements and verification procedures must apply to all practitioners who apply for appointment to the medical staff and should be as stringent and thorough as a hospital's.

2. *Verify credentials through primary sources*. It is important that the facility get primary-source verification. Documents in the credential files can be copies, but the authenticity of those copies must have been verified by the organization holding the original.

3. *Use peer letters to verify credentials.* Many centers rely on peer letters—often from a hospital where a practitioner practices—to check competency and conduct a quality review. That's acceptable, but these organizations should consider developing a form letter to help ensure that such surveys are consistent and comprehensive.

4. *Develop a quality review committee.* Anesthesiologists (and other practitioners with anesthesia and/or conscious sedation privileges) should have relevant performance and outcomes data reviewed by a committee. The results of these reviews should affect decisions regarding appointment and reappointment.

Privileging in ambulatory centers

Because practitioners who provide anesthesia care (or other services) may perform different procedures in a hospital than in an ambulatory setting, their privileges must be facility-specific and reflective of the care they will actually provide at the facility in question. Independent ambulatory centers must not carry over privileges granted by an unaffiliated hospital—or vice versa. Nor should a freestanding ambulatory center assume that, because a practitioner was granted specific privileges by a hospital, he or she is competent to perform the same or similiar procedures at the center. Practitioners must submit separate requests for privileges to each organization, and the organizations must evaluate each application separately and with equal care.

Furthermore, privileges should be practitioner-specific—especially for risky or advanced procedures. Since different practitioners have different levels of competence, organizations place patients at risk if they grant privileges simply because a practitioner has completed a specific residency training program. An anesthesiologist might be qualified to participate in many operative procedures, but not in open heart surgery or in pediatric surgery. While it's becoming more acceptable to grant a specific set of "core privileges" to all practitioners in a clinical department, organizations must evaluate carefully the ability of practitioners to perform the procedures for which they request privileges.

Anesthesia care by nonphysician providers

There are approximately 24,000 certified registered nurse anesthetists in the United States. It is estimated they participate in delivery of 65 percent of the anesthetics administered to patients each year—most frequently as part of an anesthesia care team overseen by an anesthesiologist. To participate in the treatment of patients, CRNAs should have the following:

- certification by the AANA Council on Certification of Nurse Anesthetists;
- current state licensure as a registered nurse; and
- current professional liability insurance.

It is important that the work of CRNAs be consistent with state and federal mandates, as well as with the institution's bylaws and rules and regulations. At times, anesthesiologists will necessarily supervise or direct CRNAs; in some situations, other licensed independent practitioners—such as surgeons, dentists (see Exhibit 5), or podiatrists—may supervise. If CRNAs are working without supervision or medical direction, it is important that state law and institutional policies allow them

Exhibit 5	Granting dentistry privileges

According to the American Dental Association (ADA), the clinical privileges required for administering local and general anesthesia in dental practice should be "consistent with the policies of the medical staff of the individual's hospital and in conformance with state practice act policies" (January 1995, "Guidelines for the Delineation of Clinical Privileges in Dentistry"). Dentists who administer anesthesia (who have a DMD or DDS doctoral degree) are certified by the National Board of Anesthesiology (NBA), which examines trained dentists who have completed an ACGME-accredited program and who are working at hospitals. The NBA requirements for certification are:

- graduate of an approved dental school;
- valid license to practice dental anesthesiology;
- conformance with standards of code of ethics;
- completion of full-term, ACGME-accredited residency in anesthesiology;
- verification of performance on own initiative of 200-plus anesthetic procedures;
- verification of staff privileges in anesthesiology; and
- two recommendations from NBA, ABA, or AOBA diplomates.

to do so. The JCAHO does not require that an anesthesiologist supervise CRNAs, only that:

- the activity of CRNAs be consistent with state laws and the rules of the healthcare facility; and
- the quality of care provided by CRNAs, anesthesiologists, and any other authorized practitioner be comparable.

Developing policies on credentialing and privileging

To be effective, policies that address credentialing and privileging requirements for practitioners that provide anesthesia and conscious sedation must take the following issues into account:

- state law;
- the medical needs of the facility's patient population; and
- the organization's mission and vision.

The policy must also address the minimum practitioner qualifications, scope of practice, and, if relevant, requirements regarding the supervision of nonphysician practitioners.

Performance improvement and peer review

The JCAHO requires the medical staff to be involved in performance improvement initiatives and assume a leadership role in improving the level of care. Therefore, LIPs who administer anesthesia need to participate in relevant peer-review sessions, and they must work with PI teams seeking to improve the quality of anesthesia care and related services.

Continuing medical education

Hospitals and ambulatory care centers generally do not require anesthesia practitioners to take part in more continuing medical education (CME) than is mandated by licensing bodies—although the JCAHO expects facilities to consider a practitioner's CME record during the reappointment process. Furthermore, healthcare facilities rarely develop internal CME programs and curricula. In choosing CME programs, therefore, anesthesia practitioners should ensure that the courses are approved by the American Medical Association—or, in the case of CRNAs, the American Nurses Association.

The JCAHO Survey

Editor's note: Although the basic agenda and structure of JCAHO surveys are usually quite uniform, each organization's survey experience tends to vary. Individual surveyors emphasize different issues, depending on their own areas of expertise and on the range of services offered by an organization or facility. This variability makes it a challenge to tell all organizations exactly what to expect during a JCAHO survey. Rather than do so here, the author has chosen to introduce organizations to key aspects of the survey process by profiling briefly one hospital's experience and observations.

Jan Magallanez, RN, entered the room like she was coming home. And why not? Magallanez, then the coordinator for regulatory compliance for St. Joseph's Hospital and Medical Center at Mercy Healthcare Arizona, had a *Comprehensive Accreditation Manual for Hospitals* under one arm and a stack of hospital policies and procedures under the other, and she was about to talk about JCAHO surveys. She was on familiar ground. A veteran of many JCAHO surveys, who's also logged many years of service in quality improvement, Magallanez is uniquely qualified to discuss the survey process—both generally and as it pertains to anesthesia-related standards.

"If you leave here understanding only one thing about JCAHO surveys and survey prep," she said as she bustled into the room, "let it be this: Know your policies and procedures; know your bylaws, your protocols, and your rules and regulations. Study these documents carefully when you're preparing for a survey. JCAHO surveyors will, and they will hold you to them."

Much of the advice that follows, whether it's in direct quotes or not, was gleaned from an in-depth discussion of the survey process with Magallanez.

The survey process

The JCAHO's survey team for hospitals usually includes a nurse, a physician, and an administrator—although this depends on the number of beds in a facility and the range of services it provides. The JCAHO may send more surveyors to very large facilities and fewer to very small facilities. Hospital surveys typically last three days, but can take anywhere from two to five days, with the size of the facility again being the key determining factor.

A person with a background in healthcare administration and a physician usually survey ambulatory facilities. Typical ambulatory surveys last two or three days, but may take longer for organizations with multiple sites or facilities separated by large distances. Surveyors might not visit every site in an ambulatory network, but it's worth noting that, according to JCAHO documents, they always visit every site that offers anesthesia services.

How is anesthesia competence assessed?

JCAHO surveyors could address anesthesia-related standards during many survey sessions (see Figure 4.1). Facilities, therefore, must be prepared to discuss anesthesia at just about any time. However, the document review, medical records review, unit visits, and building tour are likely to be the most crucial sessions. More than any others, these sessions allow surveyors to determine whether an organization's anesthesia-related policies and procedures are consistent with all standards and regulations, and whether members of the medical and hospital staffs comply with the organization's policies and all other relevant requirements.

The opening conference

Surveys usually begin with an opening conference, which includes the survey team, the senior administrator from the facility being surveyed, and the facility staff person who is coordinating the survey agenda and activities. This conference gives all parties an opportunity to review and, if necessary, discuss revisions to the survey agenda.

The PI overview

After the opening conference, JCAHO surveyors usually begin the performance improvement overview. During this session, they will want to see evidence that your facility has a systematic, multidisciplinary program for improving performance. This is a crucial session and should include key members of senior management and physician leaders who participate in performance improvement activities. Furthermore, an organization's performance improvement plan and program should address issues related to anesthesia and conscious sedation, since

Figure 4.1

Survey sessions that address anesthesia

Performance improvement overview

Document review

Leadership interview

Unit visits, including:

- anesthetizing locations

- ambulatory/outpatient clinics

- emergency services

- imaging services

- inpatient units (for hospitals)

- pharmacy services

Medical records review

Ethics interview

Medication use and nutrition care interview

Anesthesia, operative, and other invasive procedures interview

Infection control interview

Human resources interview

Medical staff credentials interview

Patient care interview

Medical staff leadership interview

Nursing leadership interview

Building tour

these services are risky and can have a significant impact on outcomes and quality of care. Participants at the PI overview should be ready to discuss data-driven initiatives designed to improve the quality of anesthesia care—including responses to sentinel events (see page 58) that involved anesthesia or sedation.

Document and records reviews

As with the PI overview, surveyors generally hold the document review session on the first day of a survey. "The survey team will want to see your bylaws, policies and procedures, and any other functional documents your facility may have," said Magallanez. "For example, they may want to see your informed consent policy. Then they will want to see how you comply with the policy." Policies that are important in the context of anesthesia and conscious sedation include those regarding:

- informed consent;
- preanesthesia assessments;
- delineation of clinical privileges;
- provision of comparable levels of care; and
- medication use and control—especially for controlled substances.

Surveyors will review key documents during this session—such as the preanesthesia and postanesthesia assessment records, anesthesia records, and consent agreements. It often makes sense for hospitals to audit these documents in advance of a survey to identify deficiencies and improve their documentation processes as needed. "Several years ago, our hospital became concerned that some preoperative assessments lacked the actual patient weights and baseline oxygen-saturation data," Magallanez said, explaining how audits help St. Joseph's prepare for surveys. "By performing a medical records review, and through a subsequent change in the preoperative nursing assessment process, we were able to improve documentation dramatically.

"The chart review also revealed that some of our anesthesia preoperative assessments did not include a physical status classification or list medication allergies," she added. "Working through the anesthesia committee, we modified the anesthesia record and distributed educational information to the staff anesthesiologists, which helped to dramatically raise our compliance with this JCAHO expectation. We also gained an additional benefit from this process through improved documentation on informed consent for anesthesia."

During the medical records review, surveyors search for evidence that staff consistently document the following:

- preoperative history and physical;
- diagnosis;
- preanesthesia assessment;
- anesthesia plan;
- a determination by an LIP that the patient is appropriate for the anesthesia;
- a nursing care plan;
- patient re-evaluation prior to the anesthesia;
- patient monitoring during the anesthesia;
- postanesthesia monitoring; and
- patient discharge from the postanesthesia care unit by an LIP or in accordance with uniform medical staff criteria.

Unit visits

To get a first-hand look at patient care procedures, surveyors will visit wards and units to observe and speak with patients, physicians, and hospital staff. They will want to see whether staff consistently follow policies and procedures. They'll note whether staff effectively educate patients and families about anesthesia and about alternative treatment options. They'll be particularly interested to know whether staff take special educational needs into account, such as language or cultural differences. They'll also check to see whether qualified practitioners assess patients, formulate anesthesia plans, and obtain consent.

In the document and record review sessions, the JCAHO wants to see that a facility has clear guidelines for patient care during anesthesia. During unit visits, surveyors determine how well staff understand and follow these guidelines, the idea being that diligent compliance with effective policies usually translates into safe, effective anesthesia care. "When the Harvard Medical School developed its 'Standards for Intraoperative Monitoring,'" said Magallanez, "our anesthesia department quickly incorporated them into its departmental rules and guidelines. Not only did this help us comply with the JCAHO standards, our physicians and staff are convinced it resulted in better patient care."

EC interview and building tours

During interviews with staff responsible for the environment of care and during building tours, JCAHO surveyors will check whether a facility has and follows a preventive maintenance schedule for anesthesia equipment. They'll review the preventive maintenance logs, which document that medical equipment and devices are tested and inspected appropriately. They will also need to see evidence that, when a problem or malfunction exists, the situation is documented and corrected.

"During one survey," Magallanez noted, "our chairman of anesthesia was impressed that the physician surveyor focused primarily on preventive maintenance for anesthesia equipment. The surveyor wanted to see documentation for two years' worth of service and maintenance for each of the thirty machines. Fortunately, we had it, and our the records were complete, accurate, and in compliance with the JCAHO standards and manufacturer recommendations."

Surveyors will also focus on other areas of facility management. For example:

- The facility must ensure that anesthesia-care sites have adequate supplies of oxygen, and it must identify the people responsible for maintaining that supply;
- The facility must show that it handles and disposes of contaminated waste and sharp objects appropriately;
- Staff must demonstrate that they know how to respond to emergencies (fires, natural disasters, etc.) that might require them to implement evacuation plans or perform other duties and procedures that aren't part of their normal work day; and
- The facility must be able to show that it is prepared for power failures, and that back-up equipment is maintained in ways that minimize the risk to patients during an outage.

Checking for comparable levels of care

"The survey team will visit settings in the hospital where anesthesia is administered," said Magallanez. "The team will want to see how a facility meets the requirement mandating comparable levels of care." To do so, surveyors will:

- visit your pre-operative or pre-procedure holding area and ask to review procedures and documentation for history and physical examinations, preanesthesia assessments, and anesthesia plans—all of which must be completed before the patient enters the operative suite;
- look for comparable monitoring equipment, staffing, and resuscitative equipment in various settings;
- check to ensure that uniform policies govern anesthesia care and medication use across all settings; and
- look for evidence that only practitioners with appropriate privileges and training order and/or administer anesthesia and conscious sedation.

The survey team also reviews policies governing maintenance of patient-monitoring and anesthesia-delivery systems for evidence that facilities provide a comparable level of care. "Years ago, when capnometry became available in our inpatient operating rooms, this monitoring technology was not immediately in use in our outpatient surgery center," said Magallanez. "While preparing for a survey, we realized this meant we were not meeting the standard for comparable levels of care, so we took steps to provide a capnometer for each ambulatory operating room—and in x-ray rooms, the cardiac catheterization laboratory, and the MRI unit."

Magallanez also noted that providing a comparable level of care also became an issue when the hospital opened a lithotripsy unit several years ago. Patients were given anesthesia in the unit, then taken to a recovery area. However, they were not being discharged according to the same criteria used in the operating room's postanesthesia care unit (PACU). With the assistance of the head nurse from the surgical PACU, the hospital implemented uniform discharge criteria for the lithotripsy unit and operating rooms, thereby eliminating a source of variation in the provision of postanesthesia care.

C A S E   S T U D Y

Hospital develops uniform sedation policy

Editor's note: A few years ago, with a JCAHO survey approaching, officials at St. Joseph's Hospital and Medical Center in Phoenix, Arizona, realized that their facility was probably not in compliance with the JCAHO's comparable care requirements because it did not have a single policy governing sedation across the facility. In preparation for that survey, they launched an initiative to shape such a policy. The author has profiled their efforts here, to illustrate some of the benefits of effective survey preparation.

St. Joseph's Hospital and Medical Center in Phoenix, Arizona, is an urban, tertiary healthcare facility with more than 550 licensed acute beds and an active medical staff of 559 physicians. The hospital provides diagnostic or therapeutic procedures requiring anesthesia at a wide variety of locations within the facility, including:

- the eye and dental clinics;
- the MRI, CT, and radiology suites;

- the endoscopy and lithotripsy units;
- the radiation therapy department;
- the emergency room;
- the cardiac catheterization lab; and
- the ambulatory and inpatient operating departments.

Before 1994, each location listed above had a separate sedation policy. Each unit credentialed its own practitioners, developed dosage guidelines, provided oversight within its clinical areas, developed patient-monitoring and staffing guidelines, and implemented its own quality assurance and quality improvement programs.

The challenge

These location-specific policies and programs became a problem when the JCAHO developed anesthesia standards that mandate a comparable level of care throughout an organization. The hospital decided to use performance improvement (PI) tools and techniques to develop a single policy that would help them meet that comparable-care requirement.

The process

The president of the medical staff and the chairman of the medical staff's Quality Assurance Committee created a task force to develop the uniform policy and designated an anesthesiologist to chair it. Other physician members on the task force included a radiologist, a dentist, a surgeon, a pediatrician, a pediatric intensivist, a pulmonologist, a gastroenterologist, and a cardiologist. The vice president of nursing, the quality improvement coordinators for ambulatory services and case management, and the chief clinical pharmacist also served on the task force.

The task force gathered the sedation policies and dosage guidelines that existed in the facility and analyzed existing utilization and performance data for sedation. It reviewed current literature concerning sedation, including the latest usage and dosage information for sedation-related medications. The task force took into account the role of sedation in all relevant clinical specialty areas and sought input from interested medical staff members in those areas. Armed with this information, members of the task force looked for scenarios in which sedation had a reasonable chance of causing patients to lose their protective airway reflexes.

The task force developed a drug dosage guideline table that included drugs and dosages for sedation when no loss of protective reflexes was anticipated. It also developed procedures to follow when sedation was given within these guidelines and outlined requirements regarding:

- the responsibilities of physicians and nurses;
- equipment for care and resuscitation;
- patient monitoring; and
- preprocedure, intraprocedure, and postprocedure care.

The guidelines were to be applied uniformly throughout the facility, regardless of the setting or practitioner involved.

The task force also developed guidelines to govern patient care when patients had a reasonable chance of losing their protective reflexes. These were situations involving use of drugs in higher dosages or by different routes, or when unique characteristics of the patient or procedure made loss of reflexes a possibility. These guidelines, which were more stringent than those for cases when protective reflexes were less at risk, included:

- special credentialing and privileging requirements;
- a preanesthesia evaluation;
- intraoperative and postoperative monitoring and care that is comparable to that provided in an operating room; and
- uniform staffing requirements.

The guidelines also required practitioners to notify the performance improvement department of any adverse events or trends. This requirement allowed the PI staff to track performance and identify improvement opportunities and needs.

Relevant clinical departments and committees reviewed the new guidelines—including the sedation policy (see page 125) and a flow chart (see Figure 4.2) depicting the process outlined in that policy. Then, the medical executive committee and hospital board reviewed the policy and gave final approval, opening the way for facility-wide implementation.

The outcome

St. Joseph's new policy ensured comparable levels of care for patients receiving conscious sedation and anesthesia. It also established a

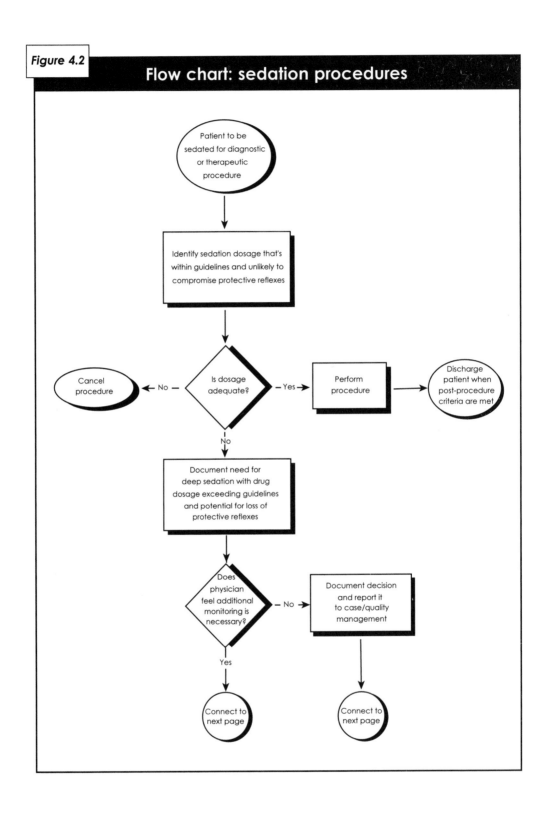

Figure 4.2

Flow chart: sedation procedures

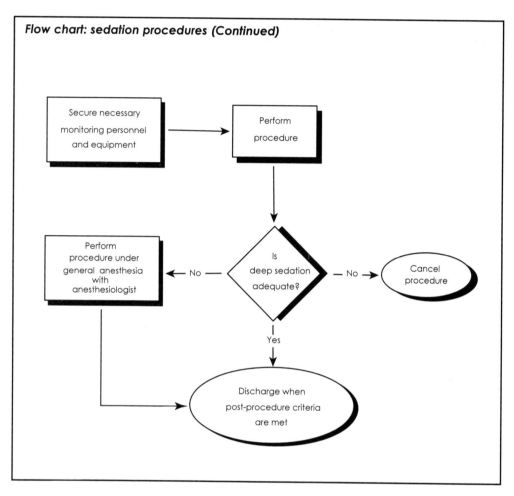

Flow chart: sedation procedures (Continued)

mechanism for identifying performance trends, adverse events, and improvement opportunities. It's worth noting that the hospital took a multidisciplinary, interdepartmental approach to developing its policy and procedures, which included the following key steps:

- The ad hoc task force incorporated suggestions and input from all clinical disciplines that rely on anesthesia or sedation;
- Relevant clinical committees reviewed the draft policy and helped create the final document; and

• The clinical committees, the medical executive committee, and the hospital board reviewed and approved the new policy.

This went a long way toward ensuring the effectiveness of the policy and procedures implemented, because it ensured that all relevant viewpoints helped shape it. It also helped St. Joseph's comply with key JCAHO requirements regarding multidisciplinary involvement in performance improvement initiatives.

Performance Monitoring and Improvement

This chapter outlines data-driven strategies for monitoring and improving the performance of practitioners involved in anesthesia care. It outlines basic quality improvement tools and techniques and discusses how a practical quality-tracking report that can help anesthesia departments build effective quality monitoring and improvement programs.

What is quality?

The term "quality" means different things to different people. To some, it implies adherence to a predetermined set of production standards. To others, it means maintaining a high level of service and customer satisfaction. Whatever your definition, monitoring and improving quality are crucial functions within healthcare organizations and should be continuous activities in the anesthesia department and any other clinical and non-clinical department whose operations affect patient care and patient safety.

What is continuous quality improvement?

Continuous quality improvement (CQI), a data-driven process for improving performance, is fueled by an open-minded, thoughtful evaluation of opportunities for change. It involves looking proactively at an organization's functions, services, and products and asking, "How can we do better?" At its most basic level, CQI is a tool for responding to existing problems, but the ideal quality-management system uses CQI techniques to prevent problems or to uncover opportunities for improving an otherwise acceptable status quo.

The terms "continuous quality improvement" and "quality assurance" (QA) are often used interchangeably. However, they are different concepts. QA involves looking for problems retrospectively. It often assumes that some amount of error or imperfection is inevitable and, therefore, acceptable. Embracing CQI means welcoming an atmosphere that encourages change and seeks it out. It means accepting the notion that processes and products can always be improved through analysis, and that each error, defect, complaint, or inefficiency—no matter how small—represents an opportunity for improvement.

Choosing quality indicators

Once a healthcare facility or an anesthesia department defines its CQI goals and expectations, it must establish reliable methods for measuring its actual performance against those goals. That means identifying quality indicators and performance criteria that are relevant to core performance expectations—your own expectations and those of patients and other "customer" groups.

Focus on "customers"
Identifying the expectations of "customers" is crucial to the selection of indicators; if you don't know what they want or need, you may monitor the wrong things and make ineffective improvement decisions. For instance, in addition to monitoring outcomes and patient safety, an

anesthesia department's CQI team might choose to monitor patient satisfaction. As part of an effort to do so, team members might track the number of patients who receive drugs to treat nausea in the postanesthesia care unit (PACU)—working under the assumption that nausea leads to dissatisfaction and that effective use of drugs to treat nausea will translate into improved satisfaction. However, if patients expect to experience some nausea following an operative procedure, they may not react to it in an overly negative way. Rather than tracking usage of anti-nausea medications, therefore, a more meaningful indicator might be the number of patients who complain about nausea. Once the frequency of complaints crosses a predetermined threshold, the CQI team might look at secondary data sets—such usage rates for drugs that treat nausea—to generate strategies for addressing the problem. But in this instance, drug usage might not be an effective primary indicator.

Identifying improvement opportunities

Once indicators have been chosen, CQI teams need to create a mechanism for organizing indicator data in meaningful ways. Fortunately, there's no need to recreate the wheel. Finance departments in many healthcare facilities use a brief report (see Figure 5.1) to monitor the financial performance of the facility. This report organizes data in a way that allows the facility to:

- compare current performance against past performance; and/or
- determine whether current performance is in line with the organization's budgeted goals and expectations.

This reporting format is particularly effective because it allows analysts to draw conclusions quickly about basic performance (to perform a

Figure 5.1

Financial performance report

Indicators	January	February	Current month	Same month last year	Budget
Avg daily census	75	74	76	76	75
Total patient days	7,000	6,800	7,100	7,300	7,000
Average length of stay	6.2	6.1	6.0	6.4	6.2
E.R. visits	1,600	1,700	1,600	1,550	1,550
Cash on hand ($)	175,000	165,000	170,000	163,000	172,000
Age of A/R (days)	56	53	53	62	55
Interest on investments (%)	10.0	9.0	9.2	15.5	10.0
Write-offs ($)	7,000	6,800	7,100	7,300	7,000
Accts receivable ($)	155,650	150,000	152,000	153,000	150,000
Accts payable ($)	75,650	79,000	62,000	78,000	65,000
Incorrect bills	18	18	16	15	N/A
Lost charges ($)	1,700	1,800	1,700	1,600	N/A

"pulse check," so to speak) while also facilitating more in-depth analysis and the formation of more sophisticated conclusions regarding performance.

Understanding the financial model

The report does not attempt to address every deficiency or problem that surfaces in a busy finance department; for instance, the steps taken to address a few incorrect bills might not appear in the report because the deficiency rate is not significant enough. Instead, the report tracks bigger-picture performance indicators—those that will demonstrate whether the facility's overall financial performance is on target. If the report suggests that the facility's financial performance is lagging, it would trigger more detailed analysis aimed at identifying potential causes and corrective actions.

Applying the financial model to anesthesia and sedation

Anesthesia departments can use this same reporting format to track performance indicators that are relevant to the provision of anesthesia and sedation—and, more importantly, to shape improvement initiatives when quality lags (see Figure 5.2). The first step, of course, involves the development of appropriate indicators that monitor the volume or frequency of key performance-related events or that reflect perceptions regarding quality and performance.

Volume indicators simply identify how often something happens. In the context of anesthesia care, such indicators might track basic procedures—for example, the total number of:

- central venous line placements;
- intraoperative blood transfusions; or
- epidural anesthetics for cesarean deliveries.

Volume indicators might also track events that are indicative of adverse events, such as:

- unexpected hospital admissions following outpatient surgery;
- instances calling for reintubation of a patient in the PACU; or
- pneumothoraces associated with placement of central venous pressure catheters.

Figure 5.2

Performance report: anesthesia & sedation

Anesthesia & Sedation

Indicators / Occurrences	Jan	Feb	Mar	Apr	May	June	July	Aug	Sept	Oct	Nov	Dec	Dept Standard
Gen'l anesthesia													
Reg'l anesthesia													
Monitored anes. care													
Sedation cases													
Sedation cases with loss of protective reflexes													
Codes responded to													
Catheter placements													
Pain mgmt. procedures													
Adverse event reports													
Patient complaints													
Practitioner complaints													
Related infections													
Late assessments													
PACU discharges by LIP													
Late H&Ps													
Related mortalities													
Poorly documented transfusions													

Performance report: anesthesia & sedation (continued)

Indicators \ Occurrences	Jan	Feb	Mar	Apr	May	June	July	Aug	Sept	Oct	Nov	Dec	Dept Standard
Perioperative myocardial infarctions													
Postdural headaches													
Patients with damaged teeth													
Patients with post-op neurological effects													
Patients with post-op pneumonia													
Patients with post-op aspiration													
Relevant malpractice claims													
Relevant delayed recoveries													
Relevant delays in surgery													
Procedure delays													
Procedure cancellation													

This second category of volume indicators correlates directly with performance quality, which makes such indicators particularly useful. However, it's also important for organizations to monitor perceptions regarding quality. This generally involves identification of indicators that gauge patient and employee satisfaction and development of vehicles (e.g., surveys, suggestion boxes, etc.) that can capture relevant data and highlight improvement opportunities.

Implementing improvement initiatives

Healthcare organizations and individual clinical departments should not treat operational changes lightly—particularly when they affect quality of care. Once improvement opportunities surface, CQI teams need to think carefully about how to act on them, and they must monitor the results of their improvement initiatives—to ensure both that they're having the effects intended and that they're not having an unexpected impact elsewhere along the continuum of care. Whenever possible, organizations may want to stage small-scale trials to test change initiatives before enacting them generally. What follows is a discussion of an structured approach to CQI that makes use of such trials.

The FOCUS PDCA approach

The FOCUS PDCA approach to quality improvement builds upon one of the earliest systematic techniques for controlling quality: the PDCA method (see Figure 5.3). Walter Shewart, a quality pioneer in manufacturing circles, developed the PDCA method in the 1920s. During the 1950s, W. Edwards Deming popularized the approach among Japanese manufacturers—which is why it is sometimes called "The Deming Cycle."

Organizations can apply Shewart's and Deming's four-stage PDCA process proactively, but most view it as a reactive tool. Rather than using the process to assess and improve systems before a problem arises, they generally wait for signs of an adverse event or outcome and apply the PDCA method in response.

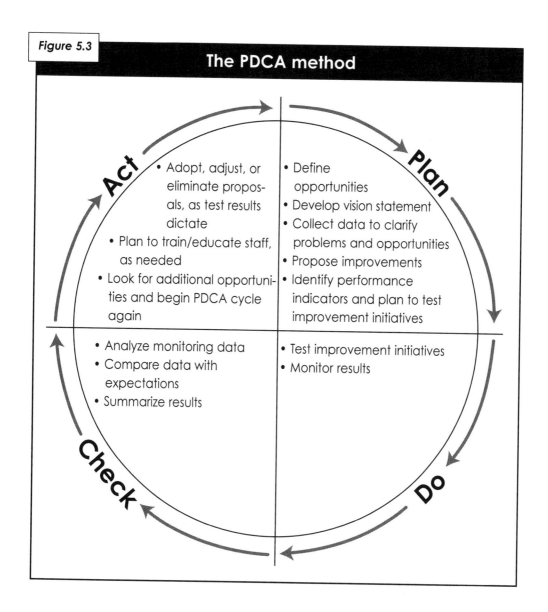

Figure 5.3

The PDCA method

Act
- Adopt, adjust, or eliminate proposals, as test results dictate
- Plan to train/educate staff, as needed
- Look for additional opportunities and begin PDCA cycle again

Plan
- Define opportunities
- Develop vision statement
- Collect data to clarify problems and opportunities
- Propose improvements
- Identify performance indicators and plan to test improvement initiatives

Check
- Analyze monitoring data
- Compare data with expectations
- Summarize results

Do
- Test improvement initiatives
- Monitor results

FOCUS PDCA (see Figure 5.4) makes the proactive potential of the basic Shewart/Deming approach more explicit. In the process, it turns an effective quality-assurance tool into a powerful vehicle for continuous quality improvement. FOCUS PDCA is founded upon the assumption that a system can always run better; it challenges organizations to seek out improvement opportunities.

FOCUS: Find a process to improve

Ideally, healthcare organizations seek to establish mechanisms that reveal systemic defects or performance variations before quality suffers dramatically—mechanisms like performance measures, monitoring systems, and an organizational culture that seeks out opportunities to change and improve. This kind of speculative analysis of anesthesia-care processes is well suited to helping department leaders and performance-monitoring teams correct systemic flaws before a serious incident puts patients, practitioners' careers, or an organization's reputation at risk.

FOCUS: Organize a team

Whether analysis teams are responsible for reactive investigation of a quality lapse or proactive identification of improvement opportunities, team members must have firsthand knowledge of the processes they are evaluating. Physicians with anesthesiology privileges, pharmacists, CRNAs, and registered nurses (especially RNs who administer sedatives and/or care for patients who receive anesthesia or sedation) should serve on CQI teams that address performance issues related to anesthesia and sedation. It also helps to involve administrative staff who understand CQI, statistical analysis, and/or the standards and regulations governing anesthesia and sedation. Finally, it's important for

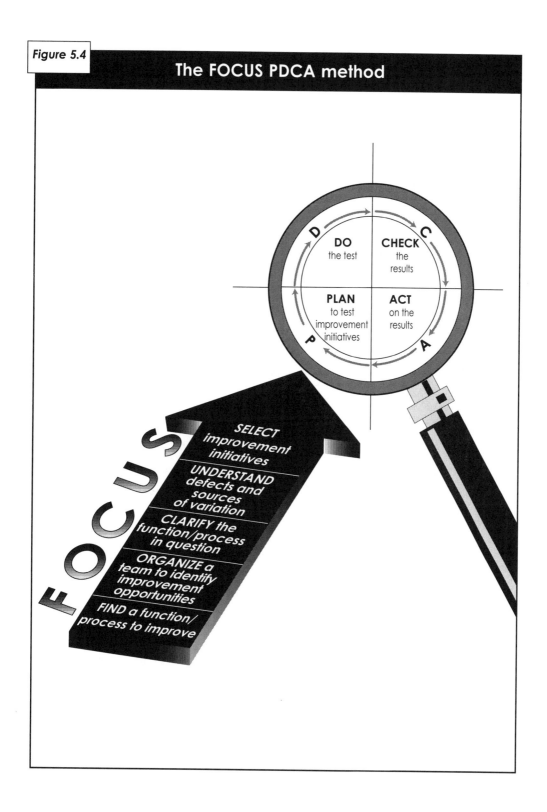

Figure 5.4

The FOCUS PDCA method

D
DO
the test

C
CHECK
the
results

PLAN
to test
improvement
initiatives

P

ACT
on the
results

A

SELECT
improvement
initiatives

UNDERSTAND
defects and
sources
of variation

CLARIFY the
function/process
in question

ORGANIZE a
team to identify
improvement
opportunities

FIND a function/
process to improve

FOCUS

CQI teams to have decision-making authority and the ability to imple-ment change, which makes the support physician and hospital leaders crucial.

FOCUS: Clarify the process in question

Once an organization has identified key processes and organized a team to improve them, that team must carefully chart each step in the processes under examination. Recruiting team members who have a relevant mix of skills and expertise is an important first step. Flow charts that diagram the processes under examination can assist in the clarification process—as can interviews with, and surveys of, others involved in the processes.

FOCUS: Understand sources of variation

Clarifying each step in the process under investigation often helps the team begin to identify gaps, inefficiencies, defects, and risk areas—aspects of that process that seem likely to prompt performance varia-tions. As they identify such flaws, it's important for team members to ask themselves what, if anything, caused them. They must peel away as many causal layers as possible to uncover the fundamental root causes of performance variation.

FOCUS: Select improvement initiatives

Once teams understand the root causes of performance variation, they can begin to propose and design improvement initiatives. If teams develop a number of improvement proposals, or if they locate more systemic defects than they can realistically address, it's important to prioritize. Team members should implement the improvement propos-als that seem most promising or likely to have the most far-reaching effects.

PDCA: Data-driven change, measurable improvement

Healthcare organizations often approach change cautiously—and they should. Not all change leads to improvement, as Coca Cola learned when it released New Coke. But, unlike miscalculations in the business sector, misguided change in healthcare can place patients' lives in jeopardy. That's why it's crucial for healthcare organizations to monitor the results of improvement initiatives. If an initiative is not having the expected effect, or if it is having unexpected impact on other functions, organizations need to react quickly—before the quality of patient care suffers significantly. The FOCUS phase of FOCUS PDCA provides a systematic, data-driven method for identifying improvement opportunities and designing change initiatives. The PDCA phase, described below, offers a proven method for implementing, evaluating, and adjusting initiatives, as needed, to make them as effective as possible.

PDCA: Plan to test/implement initiatives

Organizations often hold small-scale trials of a new process before implementing it widely. Sometimes called pilots, these test runs allow the organization to control or minimize the impact of a new method or procedure until there's clear evidence that the effects will be positive. Also, because they are limited in scope, trial runs often are more cost-effective than immediate, full-scale implementation of new policies and procedures.

Regardless of whether improvement teams choose to stage a trial, it is crucial that its members develop an action plan to guide their implementation and evaluation efforts (see Figure 5.5, page 121). Effective action plans include seven basic components:

1. a mission statement that defines a specific, measurable objective;

2. an overview of tactics (change initiatives) that will help the team fulfill its objective;

3. clear, measurable expectations regarding results;

4. identification of performance indicators to measure actual results against expectations;

5. an explanation of data-collection mechanisms to be used in monitoring those indicators;

6. designations of responsibility for each action item or tactic in the plan; and

7. a timeline for staging preliminary and final assessments of each change initiative.

The planning process should include consideration of possible direct and indirect effects of a change initiative. Patient-care functions and processes are often interconnected, but not always in obvious ways. Adjustments to one function may produce effects in others. If team members don't commit time and resources to anticipating, addressing, and monitoring such unexpected or less obvious effects, the negative results in one area could neutralize important gains in another.

PDCA: Do the test/implement change

Once the team has outlined its tactics, assigned responsibilities, and settled on a timeline for each initiative, it is ready to implement the proposed changes. Depending on the size of the team and the number of initiatives under consideration, team members may want to separate themselves into smaller work groups for this phase. If they do so, periodic meetings of the full team will help keep the overall project on

Figure 5.5

CQI Action Plan

Sample CQI action plan

Facilitator:

Launch Date:

Mission Statement:

Improvement Tactics	Performance Indicators	Data Sources & Collection Methods	Analysis Due	Results & Recommendations
tactic: coordinator: targeted result:			prelim: final:	
tactic: coordinator: targeted result:			prelim: final:	
tactic: coordinator: targeted result:			prelim: final:	
tactic: coordinator: targeted result:			prelim: final:	

track, allow work group members to seek input from others, and provide a forum for reporting and discussing preliminary findings.

PDCA: Check the results

When the trial run (or the initial phase of a full-scale implementation) is complete, the team should analyze the performance monitoring data that it collected and compare its findings against its improvement goals. Change initiatives should never go unmonitored or unanalyzed.

PDCA: Act on the results

If the results of an improvement plan are unsatisfactory, the team may need to reconsider or refine proposed changes and repeat the PDCA cycle. If, however, change initiatives meet or exceed expectations, team members should take steps to enact them across the organization. Enactment may involve working with hospital and medical staff leaders to revise existing policies and procedures, developing staff-retraining initiatives, and other activities.

Sample Sedation Policies

This appendix contains three sample policies that organizations can use as models when developing or evaluating their own policies governing sedation, conscious sedation, and/or anesthesia care.

St. Joseph's Hospital

Policy and Procedures
for Sedation and Anesthesia

1. Policy

It is the policy of St. Joseph's Hospital to provide safe and consistent care for patients receiving sedation during diagnostic and therapeutic procedures. Policy implementation is the responsibility of the practitioner ordering the sedation and the department where the sedation is administered.

These guidelines are designed to provide specific recommendations for the safe care of patients during the delivery of medications for sedation by non-anesthesiologists during diagnostic and therapeutic procedures.

2. Definitions

Sedation: The calming of an anxious, apprehensive individual through the use of drugs for which there is a reasonable expectation that, in the manner used, the sedation should not result in the loss of protective reflexes for a significant percentage of a group of patients.

Loss of protective reflexes: Loss of reflexes, including the inability to maintain a patent airway or purposeful response to physical and/or verbal stimulation as a result of a systemically administered drug.

Deep sedation: A controlled state of unconsciousness that may be accompanied by loss of protective reflexes, including inability to maintain a patent airway or purposeful response to physical and/or verbal stimulation.

3. Procedure for use of sedation within the recommended sedation dosage guidelines.[1]

3.1 Physician responsibility for use of sedation within the recommended dosage guidelines.

The physician has the responsibility for:

3.1.1 Providing the level of monitoring specified in these guidelines and to manage complications. The practitioner should be trained in and capable of providing basic life support. Training in advanced cardiac life support is strongly recommended. The responsible physician should be within immediate reach and available if problems or emergencies arise;

3.1.2 Determining that the patient is an appropriate candidate for the sedative agent to be administered. The pre-procedure evaluation should include, but not be limited to:

- the patient's history of medication allergies/reactions,
- listing of current medications and dosages,
- overall physical status,
- verifying patient compliance with pre-procedure instructions,

---

[1] *Facilities should develop sedation dosage guidelines and sedation antagonists guidelines in accordance with their specific patient populations, case mixes, and past experiences.*

A nurse or other qualified health care provider may conduct the evaluation, but final responsibility for authorization to administer the sedative rests with the physician;

3.1.3 Authorizing the administration of the sedation within the recommended sedation dosage guidelines;

3.1.4 Referring to guidelines in Section 4 of this policy in the event the sedation dosage guidelines are exceeded.

3.2 Equipment for use of sedation within the recommended sedation dosage guidelines

The department where the sedation is administered has the following equipment immediately accessible:

3.2.1 Equipment for non-invasive measurement of blood pressure;

3.2.2 A functional suction apparatus with the appropriate suction catheters;

3.2.3 Source of supplemental oxygen and the apparatus for its administration;

3.2.4 Emergency equipment including:

- Age-appropriate resuscitative supplies;
- Appropriate reversal agents.

3.3 Monitoring for use of sedation within the recommended sedation dosage guidelines

3.3.1 The sedated patient is attended during the procedure or recovery period;

3.3.2 Baseline vital signs are recorded prior to on-site sedation administration;

3.3.3 The heart rate, blood pressure, and respiratory rate are recorded every 15 minutes during the procedure. When other monitoring equipment would interfere with the procedure, pulse oximetry is required. The physician may defer the recording of monitored parameters at the 15-minute interval if such recording interferes with the diagnostic or therapeutic procedure.

3.4 Post-procedure patient care for use of sedation within the recommended sedation dosage guidelines

The patient may be transferred or discharged when the following criteria are met:

3.4.1 Vital signs are stable;

3.4.2 Patient arouses to stimuli and/or returns to pre-procedure level of consciousness;

3.4.3 Additional criteria for the patient discharged home:

- Patient mobility has been determined safe for discharge;
- A responsible person should accompany the patient home;

- Written discharge instructions should be given to the patient and/or responsible person.

4. Procedure for use of deep sedation that exceeds the recommended sedation dosage guideline

4.1 **Physician notification.** Staff will inform the responsible physician when drug doses specified in the sedation dosage guidelines are exceeded with additional doses;

4.2 **Physician evaluation.** The physician shall then evaluate the patient and determine if there will be the likelihood of loss of protective reflex. The patient's status and the determination by the physician of the need for additional monitoring is documented;

4.3 **Reporting requirements.** Staff will report to the quality improvement office all cases in which the recommended sedation dosage guidelines are exceeded and the physician determines the monitoring level for deep sedation is unnecessary;

4.4 **Loss of reflexes.** If the need for additional airway management is documented, the following deep sedation guidelines apply.

4.5 Guidelines for Deep Sedation

4.5.1 The practitioner ordering a dose of sedative exceeding the dosage specified in the sedation dosage guidelines is responsible for:

4.5.1.1 Meeting the credentialing/privileging requirements and the institutional guidelines for medication administration;

4.5.1.2 Providing total patient care including resuscitative efforts, if needed. The practitioner should be trained in and capable of providing basic life support, and have training in advanced cardiac life support, pediatric advance life support, and neonatal advance life support is strongly recommended;

4.5.1.3 Assuring the equipment and level of monitoring provided in these guidelines is available at the sedating location, including the provision of a qualified nurse (one having, at minimum, certification for basic life support and competency in required monitoring modalities) whose sole responsibility is to monitor the patient's physiologic parameters. Personnel who have advanced cardiac life support certification are immediately available, on site;

4.5.1.4 Determining that the patient is an appropriate candidate for the sedative agent to be administered. The pre-procedure evaluation should include, but not necessarily be limited to:

- the patient's history of medication allergies/reactions,
- listing of current medications and dosages,
- overall mental and physical condition,
- assessment of other medical and/or surgical problems,

A nurse or other qualified health care provider may conduct the evaluation, but final responsibility for authorization to administer the sedative rests with the physician;

4.5.1.5 Authorizing the administration of the sedation.

4.6 Pre-procedure preparation for use of deep sedation that exceeds the recommended sedation dosage guidelines

The qualified healthcare provider (see 4.5.1.1, 4.6.4) is responsible for:

4.6.1 Verifying the patient's adherence to pre-procedure instructions and reporting non-compliance to the physician;

4.6.2 Determining the presence of a responsible person who will accompany the patient home;

4.6.3 Establishing a patent intravenous line to be maintained from the beginning of medication administration until post-procedure discharge criteria are met;

4.6.4 Meeting the licensing requirements and institutional guidelines for such medication administration;

A registered nurse acts in accordance with the Arizona State Nursing Board advisory opinion.

4.7 Equipment for deep sedation exceeding recommended sedation dosage guidelines

The following equipment is immediately accessible and readily available:

4.7.1 A positive-pressure oxygen delivery system, capable of administering greater than 90% oxygen for at least 60 minutes;

4.7.2 A functional suction apparatus with the appropriate suction catheters;

4.7.3 Emergency cart with defibrillator and age-appropriate supplies;

4.7.4 Equipment for non-invasive measurement of blood pressure, pulse oximetry, and continuous electrocardiogram display.

4.8 Monitoring for deep sedation exceeding recommended sedation dosage guidelines

4.8.1 Baseline vital signs are recorded prior to sedation administration and IV access is verified;

4.8.2 A qualified registered nurse, whose sole responsibility is to monitor the patient's status, records the heart rate, blood pressure, respiratory rate and oxygen saturation every 5 minutes during the procedure. At the discretion of the attending physician, one of these four monitoring parameters may be deferred if such monitoring interferes with the diagnostic or therapeutic procedure;

4.8.3 All pertinent events taking place during the induction of, maintenance of, and emergence from deep sedation should be documented.

4.9 Post-procedure care of the patient receiving deep sedation exceeding recommended sedation dosage guidelines

4.9.1 Nursing personnel with training in resuscitation shall observe the patient post procedure. The patient's heart rate, blood pressure, respiratory rate and oxygen saturation will be continuously monitored and recorded every 15 minutes until the patient is fully awake and responds accordingly;

4.9.2 Nursing personnel may discharge patients who have met preset discharge criteria, which at minimum include:

4.9.2.1 Vital signs are within 15% of pre-procedure vital signs;

4.9.2.2 For the patient discharged home:

- Patient is able to take and retain fluids,
- Patient's mobility has been determined safe for discharge,
- A responsible person will accompany the patient home.

Patients not meeting the discharge criteria must be evaluated by a physician for disposition and proper documentation of the discharge noted.

4.10 Quality improvement

Each location administering sedation exceeding the recommended sedation dosage guidelines will report adverse occurrences to the quality improvement office.

Source: Adapted with permission of Catholic Healthcare West–Arizona and St. Joseph's Hospital and Medical Center, Phoenix, AZ.

Turville Bay MRI Center

Conscious Sedation Policy for Adult Patients

Purpose:

- To provide safe administration of IV sedation to conscious patients by registered nurse.

- To minimize physical discomfort or pain.

Equipment:

- A positive-pressure, oxygen-delivery system

- A functional suction apparatus with appropriate suction catheters

- Pulse Oximeter

- An emergency cart must be immediately accessible. This cart must contain equipment to resuscitate patients who are unconscious, have no pulse, and have stopped breathing.

Policy:

A. Personnel

1. A licensed RN must accompany the patient to and from the MRI suite and remain with the patient during the entire procedure.

2. The RN is responsible for administering drugs for sedation, monitoring patients as outlined in the guidelines that follow, managing complications, and communicating with physicians.

3. The RN must be trained in and capable of providing basic life support (at minimum). Training in advanced life support is strongly encouraged.

B. Before sedation

1. The attending physician shall provide written orders regarding the type and amount of drug to be used and the route of administration.

C. Dietary precautions

1. The use of sedation must be preceded by an evaluation of food and fluid intake.

2. No milk or solids for 8 hours before scheduled procedure.

D. Documentation at time of sedation

1. Before sedation, a health evaluation shall be performed by an appropriate licensed practitioner, which should include the following:
   a. Age and weight
   b. Health history, including:
     1) allergies
     2) drug use
     3) relevant diseases and physical abnormalities
     4) summary of previous relevant hospitalizations
     5) history of sedation or general anesthesia and any complications

6) relevant family history

c. Review of systems

d. Vital signs, including heart rate, blood pressure, respiratory rate, and temperature.

e. Physical exam, including an evaluation of the airway.

The current hospital record may suffice for adequate documentation of pre-sedation health. However, a brief note shall be written documenting that the chart was reviewed, positive findings were noted, and a management plan was formulated.

E. Documentation during treatment

1. Patient's level of consciousness and responsiveness

2. Heart rate

3. Blood pressure

4. Respiratory rate

5. Oxygen saturation

6. Name, route, site, time, dosage, and patient effect of administered drugs

7. Inspired concentrations of oxygen used

8. Adverse events

F. Documentation after treatment

1. Time and condition of patient at time of discharge from MRI suite

2. The protocol for monitoring patient at time of discharge will be per hospital policy.

G. Adverse events

1. For low oxygen saturation (less than 90% with supplemental oxygen), RN should contact attending physician ordering sedation, refrain from giving any more sedatives, and provide necessary basic life support until physician orders are received.

   a. If low saturation is secondary to airway obstruction, RN should provide chin lift-head tilt, insert oral or nasal airway, and perform bag and mask ventilation if necessary.

   b. If low saturation is secondary to benzodiazepine/narcotic overdose, Flumazenil or Naloxone may be given in accordance with the attending physician's orders.

   c. If low saturation continues despite above maneuvers, Respiratory Therapy and Anesthesia should be called to evaluate need for endotracheal intubation.

   d. In event of cardiac arrest, RN should call Code Blue in accordance with hospital policy.

Adapted slightly and reprinted by permission of Turville Bay MRI Center, Madison, WI.

Conscious Sedation Policy

Conscious sedation is the administration of drugs to dull or reduce a patient's pain and awareness without the loss of defensive reflexes (e.g., cough and gag) for the purpose of performing an invasive or non-invasive procedure.

Policy

Each patient who receives conscious sedation requires continuous cardiac monitoring and oximetry. A qualified registered professional nurse—with current basic cardiac life support and advanced cardiac life support certification—must be present to observe the patient.

Only a qualified physician who meets the criteria set by the medical executive committee may administer conscious sedatives in approved locations.

In the event that anesthesia or conscious sedation must be administered outside an approved setting, the anesthesiology department director or the covering anesthesiologist must be notified to arrange a safe alternative setting for the procedure.

Before initiating conscious sedation, emergency equipment—including oxygen pulse oximeter and code cart—must be available where the procedure will be performed. In addition, a qualified RN must be present to continuously monitor and assess the patient.

Pre-Procedure Responsibilities

Physician

1. Obtains appropriate informed consent.

2. Completes appropriate pre-operative documentation indicating that the patient is appropriate for that type of anesthesia, including a description of the patient's physical status and the plan for anesthesia (e.g., IV sedation with monitoring, medical diagnosis, risks of the procedure, etc.).

3. Schedules patient for the procedure in an approved anesthesia location.

RN

1. Verifies appropriate informed consent.

2. Gathers emergency equipment before procedure and/or induction of conscious sedative.

3. Assesses the patient's vital signs—baseline blood pressure, heart rate, respiratory rate, heart rhythm, oxygen saturation, level of consciousness, and Aldrete score—and documents the measurements.

Intra-Procedure Responsibilities

RN

1. Monitors and documents the patient's vital signs every five minutes or more frequently as necessary.

2. Assesses the patient continuously for changes in condition and/or untoward responses or effects, and reports any of the above to the responsible physician immediately.

Post-Procedure Responsibilities

Physician

1. Documents a post-anesthesia note, including pre- and post-operative diagnoses, procedure findings, complications, and plan of care.

RN

1. Monitors and documents the patient's vital signs every five minutes until the patient's Aldrete score is equal to 10 or reaches his or her pre-procedure score.

2. Notifies the responsible physician immediately if the patient doesn't meet the criteria specified above after one hour post-procedure. (The nurse shall continue to monitor and document all of the vital signs every five to 10 minutes until the patient reaches pre-procedure condition.)

3. Completes the necessary nursing documentation, including a statement regarding the patient's disposition.

4. Follows the procedure for post-operative care of patients, when the patient attains his or her pre-procedure Aldrete score.

5. Completes appropriate forms, such as nursing progress notes, per order or post-procedure policy.

Source: Hugh Greeley and Herman Williams, MD, MPH, MBA, The Top Twenty Medical Staff Policies and Procedures (Marblehead, MA: Opus Communications, 1998), pp. 3–5.

Anesthesia Guidelines and Standards

This appendix contains standards and guidelines published by the American Society of Anesthesiologists (ASA). This information was originally published in ASA's *1999 Directory of Members* and has been reprinted with permission.

Guidelines for a Minimally Acceptable Program of Any Continuing Education Requirement

(Approved by House of Delegates October 4, 1972;
last amended October 18, 1989)

I. The program should consist of a minimum of 150 hours of approved postgraduate education every three years.

II. Approved postgraduate educational experience should include the following:

Category I (minimum 60 hours)

The Society believes that 60 hours is the minimum time that should be spent in Category I efforts. We recognize that hours of credit suggested for the subcategories below are quite appropriately subject to some degree of variation from one program to another.

A. An ACGME-accredited transitional year, residency, or fellowship should be credited at 50 hours per year for full-time training. No credit for training prior to the three-year period under consideration should be allowed.

B. Fifty credit hours should be allowed for each full academic year of education leading to an advanced degree other than the MD degree in a medical field or medically related science. Education must occur within the three-year period under consideration.

C. Continuing medical education courses should be credited on an hour-for-hour basis for the number of hours of course attendance. Approved courses should include:

1. Any formally constituted meeting, program, or course taught or sponsored by a medical school accredited by the LCME.

2. Any formally constituted meeting, program, or course sponsored by an institution or hospital accredited by the AMA or State Medical Society.

3. Any formally constituted meeting, program, or course offered nationally or locally by any of the specialty societies recognized by the AMA. This would include programs sponsored by the ASA or its component societies.

D. Thirty credit hours should be allowed for each examination in which a physician participates in the ASA Self-Evaluation Program for a potential 60 credit hours per year.

Category II (maximum 90 hours)

A. Up to 24 credit hours per year should be allowed for hours of self-education by tapes such as those of the American College of Physicians or Audio-Digest.

B. Up to 24 credit hours per year should be allowed for hours of self-education through the study of medical literature related to the specialty.

C. Up to 10 credit hours per year should be allowed for hours spent teaching anesthesiology-related sciences to medical students, graduate physicians, or allied health personnel.

D. Up to 10 credit hours per year should be allowed for hours spent in the initial preparation and publication of scientific papers.

E. Up to 10 credit hours per year should be allowed for presentation of each paper, course, or exhibit at meetings of any national, regional, or local medical group recognized by the AMA.

F. Hour-for-hour credit should be allowed for such educational activities as attendance at:

1. Medical meetings, programs, courses, or scheduled grand rounds not included in previous categories.

2. Postmortems with a pathologist.

3. Journal clubs.

The Society and its Section on Education and Research will continue to coordinate and promote the availability nationally, regionally, and locally of suitable continuing medical education activities.

The decision for the initiation of programs for required continuing education shall remain a responsibility of the component societies.

Documentation of Anesthesia Care

(Approved by House of Delegates on October 12,1988)

Documentation is a factor in the provision of quality care and is the responsibility of an anesthesiologist. While anesthesia care is a continuum, it is usually viewed as consisting of preanesthesia, perianesthesia, and postanesthesia components. Anesthesia care should be documented to reflect these components and to facilitate review.

The record should include documentation of:

I. Preanesthesia Evaluation*

    A. Patient interview to review:

        1. Medical history

        2. Anesthesia history

        3. Medication history

    B. Appropriate physical examination.

    C. Review of objective diagnostic data (e.g., laboratory and x-ray).

    D. Assignment of ASA physical status (see p. 27).

    E. Formulation and discussion of an anesthesia plan with the patient and/or responsible adult.

II. Perianesthesia (time-based record of events)

    A. Immediate review prior to initiation of anesthetic procedures:

        1. Patient reevaluation

        2. Check of equipment, drugs, and gas supply

    B. Monitoring of the patient** (e.g., recording of vital signs).

    C. Amounts of all drugs and agents used, and times given.

---

*See Basic Standards for Preanesthesia Care (Editor's note: See p. 165)

**See Standards for Basic Anesthetic Monitoring (Editor's note: See p. 151)

D. The type and amounts of all intravenous fluids used, including blood and blood products, and times given.

E. The technique(s) used.

F. Unusual events during the anesthesia period.

G. The status of the patient at the conclusion of anesthesia.

III. Postanesthesia

A. Patient evaluation on admission and discharge from the postanesthesia care unit.

B. A time-based record of vital signs and level of consciousness.

C. All drugs administered and their dosages.

D. Type and amounts of intravenous fluids administered, including blood and blood products.

E. Any unusual events, including postanesthesia or postprocedural complications.

F. Postanesthesia visits.

Standards for Basic Anesthetic Monitoring

(Approved by House of Delegates on October 21,1986 and last amended on October 21, 1998)[1]

These standards apply to all anesthesia care, although in emergency circumstances, appropriate life support measures take precedence. These standards may be exceeded at any time based on the judgment of the responsible anesthesiologist. They are intended to encourage quality patient care, but observing them cannot guarantee any specific patient outcome. They are subject to revision from time to time, as warranted by the evolution of technology and practice. They apply to all general anesthetics, regional anesthetics, and monitored anesthesia care. This set of standards addresses only the issue of basic anesthetic monitoring, which is one component of anesthesia care. In certain rare or unusual circumstances, some of these methods of monitoring may be clinically impractical, and appropriate use of the described monitoring methods may fail to detect untoward clinical developments. Brief interruptions of continual[2] monitoring may be unavoidable. Under extenuating circumstances, the responsible anesthesiologist may waive the requirements marked with an asterisk (*); it is recommended that, when this is done, it should be so stated (including the reasons) in a note in the patient's medical record. These standards are not intended for application to the care of the obstetrical patient in labor or in the conduct of pain management.

---

[1] To become effective July 1, 1999.

[2] Note that "continual" is defined as "repeated regularly and frequently in steady rapid succession," whereas "continuous" means "prolonged without any interruption at any time."

Standard I

Qualified anesthesia personnel shall be present in the room throughout conduct of all general anesthetics, regional anesthetics, and monitored anesthesia care.

Objective

Because of the rapid changes in patient status during anesthesia, qualified anesthesia personnel shall be continuously present to monitor the patient and provide anesthesia care. In the event there is a direct known hazard, e.g., radiation, to the anesthesia personnel which might require intermittent remote observation of the patient, some provision for monitoring the patient must be made. In the event that an emergency requires the temporary absence of the person primarily responsible for the anesthetic, the best judgment of the anesthesiologist will be exercised in comparing the emergency with the anesthetized patient's condition and in the selection of the person left responsible for the anesthetic during the temporary absence.

Standard II

During all anesthetics, the patient's oxygenation, ventilation, circulation, and temperature shall be continually evaluated.

Oxygenation

Objective

To ensure adequate oxygen concentration in the inspired gas and the blood during all anesthetics.

Methods

Inspired gas: During every administration of general anesthesia using an anesthesia machine, the concentration of oxygen in the patient breathing system shall be measured by an oxygen analyzer with a low oxygen concentration limit alarm in use.*

Blood oxygenation: During all anesthetics, a quantitative method of assessing oxygenation, such as pulse oximetry, shall be employed.* Adequate illumination and exposure of the patient are necessary to assess color.

Ventilation

Objective

To ensure adequate ventilation of the patient during all anesthetics.

Methods

Every patient receiving general anesthesia shall have the adequacy of ventilation continually evaluated. Quantitative clinical signs, such as chest excursion, observation of the reservoir breathing bag, and auscultation of breath sound, are useful. Continual monitoring for the presence of expired carbon dioxide shall be performed unless invalidated by the nature of the patient, procedure, or equipment. Quantitative monitoring of the volume of gas expired is strongly encouraged.*

When an endotracheal tube or laryngeal mask is inserted, its correct positioning must be verified by clinical assessment and by identification of carbon dioxide expired gas. Continual endtidal carbon dioxide analysis, in use from the time of endotracheal tube/laryngeal mask placement, until extubation/removal or initiating of transfer to a postoperative care location, shall be performed using a quantitative method such as capnography, capnometry, or mass spectroscopy.*

When ventilation is controlled by a mechanical ventilator, there shall be in continuous use a device that is capable of detecting disconnection of components of the breathing system. The device must give an audible signal when its alarm threshold is exceeded.

During regional anesthesia and monitored anesthesia care, the adequacy of ventilation shall be evaluated, at least, by continual observation of qualitative clinical signs.

Circulation

Objective
To ensure the adequacy of the patient's circulatory function during all anesthetics.

Methods
Every patient receiving anesthesia shall have the electrocardiogram continuously displayed from the beginning of anesthesia until preparing to leave the anesthetizing location.*

Every patient receiving anesthesia shall have arterial blood pressure and heart rate determined and evaluated at least every five minutes.*

Every patient receiving general anesthesia shall have, in addition to the above, circulatory function continually evaluated by at least one of the following: palpation of a pulse, auscultation of heart sounds, monitoring of a tracing of intra-arterial pressure, ultrasound peripheral pulse monitoring, or pulse plethysmography or oximetry.

Body Temperature

Objective

To aid in the maintenance of appropriate body temperature during all anesthetics.

Methods

Every patient receiving anesthesia shall have temperature monitored when clinically significant changes in body temperature are intended, anticipated, or suspected.

Guidelines for Patient Care in Anesthesiology

(Approved by House of Delegates on October 3, 1967
and last amended on October 23, 1996)

I. Definition of Anesthesiology

Anesthesiology is a discipline within the practice of medi
cine specializing in:

A. The medical management of patients who are rendered uncon
scious and/or insensible to pain and emotional stress during surgical, obstetrical, and certain other medical procedures (involves
preoperative, intraoperative, and postoperative evaluation and
treatment of these patients);

B. The protection of life functions and vital organs (e.g., brain,
heart, lungs, kidneys, liver) under the stress of anesthetic, surgical, and other medical procedures;

C. The management of problems in pain relief;

D. The management of cardiopulmonary resuscitation;

E. The management of problems in pulmonary care;

F. The management of critically ill patients in special care units.

II. Anesthesiologist's Responsibilities

Anesthesiologists are physicians who, after college, have
graduated from an accredited medical school and have successfully completed an approved residency in anesthesiology,
and, in addition, may have had additional training in critical
care medicine and pain management. Anesthesiologists'
responsibilities to patients should include:

A. Preanesthetic evaluation and treatment;

B. Medical management of patients and their anesthetic procedures;

C. Postanesthetic evaluation and treatment;

D. On-site medical direction of any nonphysician who assists in the technical aspects of anesthesia care to the patient.

III. Guidelines for Anesthesia Care

A. The same quality of anesthesia care should be available for all patients:
1. 24 hours a day, seven days a week;
2. Emergency as well as elective patients;
3. Obstetrical, medical, and surgical patients.

B. Preanesthetic evaluation and preparation means that an anesthesiologist:
1. Reviews the chart.
2. Interviews the patient to:
   a. Discuss medical history, including anesthetic experiences and drug therapy.
   b. Perform any examinations that would provide information that might assist in decisions regarding risk and management.
3. Orders necessary tests and medications essential to the conduct of anesthesia.
4. Obtains consultations as necessary.
5. Records impressions on the patient's chart.

C. Perianesthetic care means:
1. Re-evaluation of patient immediately prior to induction.
2. Preparation and check of equipment, drugs, fluids, and gas supplies.

3. Appropriate monitoring of the patient.

4. Selection and administration of anesthetic agents to render the patient insensible to pain during the procedure.

5. Support of life functions under the stress of anesthetic, surgical, and obstetrical manipulations.

6. Recording the events of the procedure.

D. Postanesthetic care means:

1. A member of the anesthesia care team remains with the patient as long as necessary.

2. Availability of adequate nursing personnel and equipment necessary for safe postanesthetic care.

3. Informing personnel caring for patients in the immediate postanesthetic period of any specific problems presented by each patient.

4. Assurance that the patient is discharged in accordance with policies established by the Department of Anesthesiology.

5. The period of postanesthetic surveillance is determined by the status of the patient and the judgment of the anesthesiolgist. (Ordinarily, when a patient remains in the hospital postoperatively for 48 hours or longer, one or more notes should appear in addition to the discharge note from the postanesthesia unit.)

IV. Additional Areas of Expertise

A. Resuscitation procedures

B. Pulmonary care

C. Critical (intensive) care

D. Diagnosis and management of pain

E. Trauma and emergency care

V. Quality Assurance

The anesthesiologist should participate in a planned program for evaluation of quality and appropriateness of patient care and resolving identified problems.

Standards For Postanesthesia Care

(Approved by House of Delegates on October 12, 1988
and last amended on October 19, 1994)

These Standards apply to postanesthesia care in all locations. These
Standards may be exceeded based on the judgment of the responsible
anesthesiologist. They are intended to encourage quality patient care,
but cannot guarantee any specific patient outcome. They are subject to
revision from time to time as warranted by the evolution of technology
and practice. *Under extenuating circumstances, the responsible anesthesiologist may waive the requirements marked with an asterisk (*); it
is recommended that, when this is done, it should be so stated (including the reasons) in a note in the patient's medical record.*

Standard I

All patients who have received general anesthesia, regional anesthesia,
or monitored anesthesia care shall receive appropriate postanesthesia
management.[1]

1. A Postanesthesia Care Unit (PACU) or an area that provides
   equivalent postanesthesia care shall be available to receive
   patients after anesthesia care. All patients who receive anesthesia
   care shall be admitted to the PACU or its equivalent except by
   specific order of the anesthesiologist responsible for the patient's
   care.

2. The medical aspects of care in the PACU shall be governed by
   policies and procedures that have been reviewed and approved
   by the Department of Anesthesiology.

---

1 Refer to *Standards of Post Anesthesia Nursing Practice 1992,* published by ASPEN, for issues of nursing
care.

3. The design, equipment, and staffing of the PACU shall meet the requirements of the facility's accrediting and licensing bodies.

Standard II

A patient transported to the PACU shall be accompanied by a member of the anesthesia care team who is knowledgeable about the patient's condition. The patient shall be continually evaluated and treated during transport with monitoring and support appropriate to the patient's condition.

Standard III

Upon arrival in the PACU, the patient shall be re-evaluated and a verbal report provided to the responsible PACU nurse by the member of the anesthesia care team who accompanies the patient.

1. The patient's status upon arrival in the PACU shall be documented.
2. Information concerning the preoperative condition and the surgcal/anesthetic course shall be transmitted to the PACU nurse.
3. The member of the Anesthesia Care Team shall remain in the PACU until the PACU nurse accepts responsibility for the nursing care of the patient.

Standard IV

The patient's condition shall be evaluated continually in the PACU.

1. The patient shall be observed and monitored by methods appropriate to the patient's medical condition. Particular attention should be given to monitoring oxygenation, ventilation, circulation, and temperature. During recovery from all anesthetics, a quantitative method of assessing oxygenation, such as pulse oximetry, shall be employed in the initial phase of recovery.* This is not intended for application during the recovery of the

obstetrical patient in whom regional anesthesia was used for labor and vaginal delivery.

2. An accurate written report of the PACU period shall be maintained. Use of an appropriate PACU scoring system is encouraged for each patient on admission, at appropriate intervals prior to discharge, and at the time of discharge.

3. General medical supervision and coordination of patient care in the PACU should be the responsibility of an anesthesiologist.

4. There shall be a policy to assure the availability in the facility of a physician capable of managing complications and providing cardiopulmonary resuscitation for patients in the PACU.

Standard V

A physician is responsible for the discharge of the patient from the postanesthesia care unit.

1. When discharge criteria are used, they must be approved by the Department of Anesthesiology and the medical staff. They may vary depending upon whether the patient is discharged to a hospital room, to the Intensive Care Unit, to a short stay unit, or home.

2. In the absence of the physician responsible for the discharge, the PACU nurse shall determine that the patient meets the discharge criteria. The name of the physician accepting responsibility for discharge shall be noted on the record.

Basic Standards for Preanesthesia Care

(Approved by House of Delegates on October 14, 1987)

These standards apply to all patients who receive anesthesia or moni-tored anesthesia care. Under unusual circumstances, e.g., extreme emergencies, these standards may be modified. When this is the case, the circumstances shall be documented in the patient's record.

Standard I

An anesthesiologist shall be responsible for determining the patient's medical status, developing an anesthesia plan, and acquainting the patient or the responsible adult with the proposed plan.

Development of an appropriate plan of ansthesia care is based upon:

1. Reviewing the medical record.
2. Interviewing and examining the patient to:
    a. Discuss the medical history, previous anesthestic experiences, and drug therapy.
    b. Assess those aspects of the physical condition that might affect decisions regarding perioperative risk and management.
3. Obtaining and/or reviewing tests and consultations necessary to the conduct of anesthesia.
4. Determining the appropriate prescription of preoperative medica-tions as necessary to the conduct of anesthesia.

The responsible anesthesiologist shall verify that the above has been properly performed and documented in the patient's record.

Guidelines for Delineation of Clinical Privileges in Anesthesiology

(Approved by House of Delegates on October 15, 1975 and last amended on October 21, 1998)

The following guidelines are designed to assist anesthesiologists and organizations in developing a program for the delineation of clinical privileges in anesthesiology. The guidelines are meant to apply to physicians practicing anesthesiology within an organization that has a formal process for delineating privileges and a program of peer review that evaluates the clinical performance and patient care results of physicians who are granted clinical privileges in anesthesiology.

Anesthesiology is the practice of medicine. Clinical privileges in anesthesiology are granted to physicians who are qualified by training to render patients insensible to pain and to minimize stress during surgical, obstetrical, and certain medical procedures using general anesthesia, regional anesthesia, or sedation/analgesia to a level at which a patient's protective reflexes are likely to be obtunded. Performance of preanesthetic, intra-anesthetic, and postanesthetic evaluation and management are essential components of the practice of anesthesiology.

Privileges in anesthesiology should be awarded on a time-limited basis, not to exceed two years. The granting, reappraisal, and revision of clinical privileges should be in accordance with medical staff bylaws and institutional/facility rules and regulations, as applicable.

To be awarded medical staff privileges in anesthesiology, a physician must fully meet certain required criteria. It is possible to make all the following criteria mandatory or to have a mixture of required and optional criteria. Organizations should determine which criteria to include and whether to include additional criteria based on the institution's individual requirements and preferences. For example, some facilities may decide that certification by the American Board of Anesthesiology is a requirement for clinical privileges in anesthesiology, while others may deem board certification to be desirable but not essential. Similarly, some institutions may decide that subspecialty fellowship training is needed for certain clinical privileges, while others may not. Some organizations may wish to recognize residency training obtained or certification awarded outside the United States. Institutions granting subspecialty clinical privileges may wish to recognize experience as an alternative to formal training in a subspecialty of anesthesiology. Some institutions may wish to modify certain requirements for physicians who have recently completed their residency or fellowship training.

Criteria to be considered for delineation of clinical privileges in anesthesiology education:

- Graduation from a medical school accredited by the Liaison Committee on Medical Education (LCME), from an osteopathic medical school or program accredited by the American Osteopathic Association (AOA), or from a foreign medical school that provides medical training acceptable to and verified by the Educational Commission on Foreign Medical Graduates (ECFMG).
- Completion of an anesthesiology residency training program approved by the Accreditation Council for Graduate Medical Education (ACGME) or by the AOA.

- Permanent certification by the American Board of Anesthesiology (ABA) or current recertification within the time interval required by the ABA.
- Current Physician's Recognition Award of the American Medical Association or completion of 100 hours of continuing medical education (CME) over two years, of which 40 hours are in Category I of the Accreditation Council for Continuing Medical Education (ACCME).
- Compliance with relevant state or institutional requirements for CME.
- At least 50 percent of CME hours in the primary specialty of practice.
- Certificate indicating completion of a course in advanced life support within 24 months preceding application for clinical privileges.

The following items are for organizations granting physicians clinical privileges to practice in a subspecialty of anesthesiology:

- Completion of a fellowship approved by the ACGME (critical care medicine, pain medicine, pediatric anesthesia) or by the AOA, or a fourth clinical year (CA-4) or fellowship of at least 12 months' duration not accredited by the ACGME or by the AOA (e.g., obstetric or cardiac anesthesia).
- Current ABA certification in pain management (certificate of added qualifications in pain management) or in critical care medicine (certificate of special qualifications in critical care medicine).

Licensure

- Current, active, unrestricted medical or osteopathic license in a United States state, district, or territory of practice. (Exception: Physicians employed by the federal government may have a current active medical or osteopathic license in any US state, district, or territory.)
- Current, unrestricted DEA registration (schedules II-V) or no history of revocation of DEA registration (schedules II-V) within the past five years.
- No disciplinary action (final judgments) against any medical or osteopathic license or by any federal agency, including Medicare/Medicaid, in the last five years.

Performance Improvement

- Member of an organization that conducts peer review of its members.
- Active participation in an ongoing process that evaluates clinical performance and patient care results of the physician through continuous quality improvement (CQI).

Personal Qualifications

- Agreement in writing to abide by the ASA "Guidelines for the Ethical Practice of Anesthesiology." *(Editor's note: These guidelines can be found in the American Society of Anesthesiologists' 1999 Directory of Members, pp. 470-1.)*
- No report of any adjudicated violation of ASA "Guidelines for the Ethical Practice of Anesthesiology" or of any adjudicated ethical violation reported by any medical society or medical or osteopathic licensing organization.
- Membership in a county, state, or national medical association

or in a state or national specialty society that requires members to subscribe to the AMA Principles of Medical Ethics or to the ASA "Guidelines for the Ethical Practice of Anesthesiology."

- Certification in writing that "I am in good health and have no physical or mental limitation, including alcohol or drug use, that could impair my ability to render quality patient care."

- No record of any felony or fraud conviction.

Practice Pattern

- Site of practice is in an office, clinic, or hospital currently accredited by the Joint Commission on Accreditation of Healthcare Organizations (JCAHO) or by the Accreditation Association for Ambulatory Health Care (AAAHC), or that complies with the ASA "Guidelines for Ambulatory Anesthesia and Surgery." (Editor's note: These guidelines can be found in the American Society of Anesthesiologists' 1999 Directory of Members, pp. 465-6.)

- Malpractice claims experience (based on final judgments)— risk-adjusted for frequency and severity with respect to specialty, years in practice, and jurisdiction of practice—that is judged acceptable by the institution's medical staff or peer review group.

- No record of disciplinary action in the National Practitioner Data Bank (NPDB) within the last five years.

- Scope and quality of clinical skills, as evidenced by ongoing peer review, that are deemed appropriate by the organization granting clinical privileges.

Sample Educational Material

This appendix contains the slightly adapted text of an educational brochure that Scottsdale North Anesthesiologists, PLC, uses to educate patients and their families about anesthesia care and sedation. This text is the property of Scottsdale North Anesthesiologists, PLC, and was reprinted with permission.

About Your Anesthesia

Editor's note: The following text was developed by an anesthesia group practice for an educational brochure for patients. It is a good example of how anesthesia practitioners can use explanatory materials to educate patients and their families about anesthesia and, thereby, ensure patients are less anxious and better prepared to undergo treatment.

About your anesthesiologist

Each of our anesthesiologists is a medical doctor (MD) who is a trained specialist for administering a wide range of anesthetics and anesthesia services. Some of our anesthesiologists have additional specialized anesthesia training in pediatric anesthesia, neuro-anesthesia and cardiovascular anesthesia.

Your anesthesiologist will meet with you just before surgery

We will review your medical history and ask you about any medication allergies, past operations, and any health history factors or past experiences that may influence your anesthesia. We will discuss the anesthesia you will be receiving. Your anesthetic will be tailored to meet your needs for comfort throughout surgery. You can rest assured that your personal safety and comfort is a priority.

Your anesthesiologist spends all of his/her time during the surgical procedure ensuring your safety. The risks associated with anesthesia have been vastly reduced with new monitoring equipment. Any significant changes in blood pressure, heart rate, or other vital functions are treated immediately. The medications are used very carefully to make sure that your surgical experience is as pleasant as possible. The association of nausea after anesthesia has been significantly decreased with newer medications.

What type of anesthesia should you have?

The type of anesthesia you will require is dependent upon the surgery you are going to have. In most cases, your surgeon requests that we use a certain type of anesthesia that he/she feels will give you the greatest degree of comfort throughout the surgery.

Many operations require a general anesthetic, while others can be performed with a regional block, spinal anesthesia, or intravenous sedation.

Going to the operating room is not a normal experience

Your surgeon, anesthesiologist, and the entire surgical staff recognize the natural anxiety with which most patients approach surgery. We believe a description of the type of anesthesia helps patients to prepare for it.

General anesthesia

When general anesthesia is used, you will sleep throughout the operation with absolutely no pain or discomfort. You will be sound asleep and under the care of your anesthesiologist throughout surgery.

Once you are settled on the operating table, to ensure your maximum safety, you will be connected to several monitors, which your anesthesiologist will loosely watch throughout surgery. A blood pressure cuff will be placed around your arm (or leg) so that your blood pressure can be monitored. EKG pads will be attached so that your heart recording can be continuously monitored. You will be connected to an oximeter, which records the amount of oxygen in your blood. Other monitors are used to gauge your response to medications. After you have breathed in oxygen with a mask for a few minutes, a quick acting sedative will be given through the intravenous tubing.

The anesthetic gas that you will breathe and other medications (given through the intravenous catheter) will keep you asleep and pain free. Once you are asleep, we will adjust the medication for your size and your response to the administered dose. We will continuously monitor your blood pressure, pulse, EKG, and the amount of oxygen in your blood and will remain by you throughout surgery for your comfort and safety. After your surgery, we will accompany you to the recovery room.

IV sedation with local anesthesia

When intravenous anesthesia is used, you will be sedated and under the care of your anesthesiologist throughout the operation. Once you are settled on the operating table, you will be connected to several monitors.

A quick acting sedative will be given through the intravenous tubing after you have breathed pure oxygen for a few minutes. Once you are sedated, we will adjust the medication for your size, your level of anxiety, and your response to the administered dose. The level of anesthesia will allow you to rest comfortably throughout your surgery. You might feel some discomfort while the local anesthetic is being injected into the surgical site by your surgeon. Once the local anesthetic has been injected, you should not experience further discomfort.

Spinal anesthesia and regional block

If you are having a spinal anesthetic or regional block, your anesthesiologist will discuss the procedure with you preoperatively.

Important things to remember

Any medication that you are taking on a regular basis should be taken on the morning of surgery with a sip of water *unless* you are instructed differently by your surgeon.

Adults should not eat or drink anything for 8 hours before surgery. Unless otherwise directed by your surgeon, please do not eat or drink anything after midnight the night before your surgery. This means absolutely nothing by mouth—not even water, ice chips, coffee or tea, mints, chewing gum, tablets, lollipops, candy, or any other substance. You may have a sip of water when taking any required medications.

If your surgery is scheduled for 2:00 PM or later, you may have clear liquids, juice, or water for breakfast. Please do *not* have milk or drinks containing caffeine, such coffee or tea.

For children under age 12 and infants, please follow *your* surgeon's advice on eating and drinking before surgery.

High blood pressure, if it is under control, will not prevent you from having successful surgery. Please ask your surgeon about taking your normal antihypertensive medication on the morning of your surgery with a sip of clear water only.

Your blood pressure may become elevated during surgery because of medications given or because of stress. Should this occur, medications are available and will be given intravenously to safely reduce your blood pressure.

If you have diabetes that requires insulin, your surgeon (or your anesthesiologist) will give you instructions about taking a reduced dose of insulin on the morning of surgery. Unless your surgeon instructs you on your insulin dose for the day of surgery, you will need to contact your anesthesiologist a few days before surgery. During surgery and the recovery period, we may extract a few drops of blood from your finger to check your blood sugar level and then make any needed adjustments in insulin dosage.

The goals of your anesthesiology team:
- Treat each patient the way we would want to be treated if we were patients
- Patient safety
- Patient comfort
- Patient privacy
- Make your surgical experience as pleasant as possible

Throughout surgery, your anesthesiologist will:
- Monitor your pulse and blood pressure
- Monitor the oxygen in your blood
- Monitor your response to medications
- Adjust medications to your size and your response to medication

After surgery, your anesthesiologist will:
- Accompany you to the recovery room.
- Assure your comfort in the recovery room and administer any medications that will make you more comfortable.

Insurance billing

We will bill your insurance company for our anesthesiology services for those procedures covered by your health insurance policy. You will be responsible for any necessary co-payment, deductible, or charges not covered. For those procedures not covered by any health insurance policy, payment is requested one week before the day of surgery.

Anesthesia charges for cosmetic or aesthetic plastic surgery

Aesthetic or cosmetic plastic surgery is not covered by a health insurance plan. To reserve our services, we request that payment for anesthesiology services be made one week before the day of surgery. Mastercard, VISA, money order, or a cashier's check are accepted. Personal checks are not accepted. If the planned surgical procedure extends past our scheduled time, we will bill you the additional usual and customary amount for our services.

Anesthesia charges for infertility surgery

When applicable, we will bill your insurance company for anesthesiology services related to these procedures. You will be responsible for any necessary co-payment, deductible, or charges not covered. Many infertility procedures are not covered by health insurance.

For procedures that are not covered by insurance, we request that payment for anesthesiology services be made one week before the day of surgery. Mastercard, VISA, money order, or a cashier's check are accepted. Personal checks are not accepted. If the planned surgical procedure extends past our scheduled time, we will bill you the additional usual and customary amount for our services.

Adapted by permission of Scottsdale North Anesthesiologists, PLC

Related Products from Opus Communications, The Greeley Company, and The Greeley Education Company

Books

The Compliance Guide to the Medical Staff Standards: Winning Strategies for Your JCAHO Survey, Second Edition

by Richard E. Thompson, MD

The Compliance Guide to the Medical Staff Standards: Winning Strategies for Your JCAHO Survey, Second Edition simplifies your survey preparation efforts and even teaches you how to preserve those efforts after your survey. It explains and examines the JCAHO medical staff standards and offers advice on how to

- avoid common mistakes that can adversely affect JCAHO accreditation;
- complete survey preparation tasks that will help you gather information, share it, and use it to plan for improvement;
- review your hospital's current preparation activities for the medical staff using the provided checklists; and
- share information on the medical staff standards with medical staff leaders, the hospital's survey coordinator, and physician leaders.

Comprised of over 150 pages, containing forms, checklists, and examples, this guidebook examines the 1998 medical staff standards and offers detailed advice on how to comply with them. Each chapter ranks the standards by degree of difficulty so you'll know exactly where to focus your efforts first. **($87/copy, 170 pages #MSS2N)**

The Credentialing Desk Reference: A Complete Listing of Primary Sources, Definitions, Hard-to-Find Facts, and Advice, 2000 Edition

by Jack Zusman, MD

The Credentialing Desk Reference, 2000 provides medical staff services professionals and personnel departments with the critical information they need to facilitate the credentialing and privileging process. Comprised of over 700 pages of easy-to-access, essential information for medical staff offices, personnel departments, and any individuals or groups that evaluate applicants for various health care professions, including:

- Credentialing and privileging "hot buttons"
- A current listing of schools, licensing agencies, and certifying boards for physicians, dentists, podiatrists, physician assistants, nurse-midwives, nurse anesthetists, and psychologists
- A list of more than 350 specialty associations, societies, colleges, and academies
- A listing of the main accrediting organizations for the various types of health care organizations
- A complete resource section with a listing of national and regional credentialing verification organizations (CVOs), credentialing software, and credentialing-related periodicals, books, and videos.

All listings include addresses, phone and fax numbers, internet addresses (when available), and information on fees and organization policies, where appropriate. **($247/copy, 740 pages #CDR2N)**

The Directory of Complementary and Alternative Medicine

This 400-page directory is the first comprehensive resource of its kind. It classifies and describes over 250 complementary and alternative medicine (CAM) therapies and cross references approximately 2,000 variations on those therapies. It explains, in detail, how each type of therapist should be credentialed or evaluated and includes contact information for main organizations such as training programs, certifying boards, and associations.

Each entry includes:

- A detailed description of the therapy
- Recognized titles of those who practice each therapy
- Education and training requirements
- Licensing and certification information
- Professional associations
- Practice sites
- Cross-references to related therapies
- Addresses, telephone and fax numbers, e-mail, and Web site information for over 800 alternative therapy organizations!

The Directory of Complementary and Alternative Medicine covers all major and minor complementary and alternative healing modalities, including newly emerging therapies and therapies commonly used in other cultures.
($129/copy, 400 pages, #DCAN)

First Do No Harm: A Practical Guide to Medication Safety and JCAHO Compliance

This book examines important new strategies for improving the safety of medication use—strategies that are transforming the way the healthcare industry thinks about over-all patient safety. It includes a thorough discussion of the JCAHO's sentinel event policy, and it offers advice on complying with JCAHO standards related to medication use and sentinel events.

First Do No Harm profiles organizations that are putting landmark thinking on patient safety to use in practical, innovative ways. It discusses strategies for:

- Avoiding medication errors and other adverse drug events
- Using root-cause analysis to investigate adverse drug events and to identify systems improvements that will help prevent similar incidents
- Avoiding JCAHO Type I recommendations

Drug treatment is inherently risky, but the healthcare industry is beginning to identify and embrace strategies that may help organizations limit and manage those risks. *First Do No Harm* will help you stay on the leading edge of this industrywide transformation, and it will help your facility avoid incidents that place its patients and its reputation at risk.
($87/copy, 200 pages #MEDN)

The Greeley Guide to Medical Staff Credentialing

Designed as a step-by-step guide to credentialing medical staff applicants, this user-friendly guidebook helps you to:

- Streamline existing credentialing systems
- Select the most highly qualified providers
- Comply with the requirements of the most demanding accreditors and regulators
- Minimize the risk of legal problems—and potential litigation costs that can run into the millions
- Maintain a competitive edge in the managed care marketplace
- Ultimately improve the quality of patient care

As an added bonus, the book and its accompanying software contain over 80 easy-to-use sample policies, forms, letters, and checklists!
($127/copy, 302 pages, #MSC2N)

JCAHO Survey Coordinator's Handbook, Second Edition

Designed to walk you through the complicated survey preparation process from start to finish, *The JCAHO Survey Coordinator's Handbook* offers easy-to-understand guidelines, tips, and other valuable suggestions to help you and your organization to successfully meet JCAHO requirements.

With this handbook's practical, step-by-step advice, you'll learn how to develop a survey preparation plan, review your documents and medical records for JCAHO compliance, and prepare your staff for surveyors' questions—all within your time frame. **($97/copy, 204 pages #SCHN)**

JCAHO Mock Survey Made Simple, 1999 Edition

by Kathryn A. Chamberlain, CPHQ, Candace J. Hamner, RN, MA
Written by two JCAHO survey coordinators whose last surveys resulted in accreditation with commendation, this book is written in plain English and provides practical, easy-to-use checklists to make your mock survey a snap to coordinate. *The JCAHO Mock Survey Made Simple, 1999 Edition* has done all the legwork for you, dissecting the JCAHO's *Comprehensive Accreditation Manual for Hospitals (CAMH)* and breaking down the information into a series of manageable, user-friendly compliance checklists. In this convenient, 250-page workbook, you'll find comprehensive checklists for pinpointing problem survey areas before they turn into Type I recommendations. **($97/copy, 250 pages #JMS2N)**

Patient and Family Education: The Compliance Guide to the JCAHO Standards

by Joan Iacono, RN, MSN, MBA, and Ann Campbell, RN, MSN
Patient and Family Education: examines the current patient and family education (PF) and related standards for hospitals and explains them in simple, practical terms. You will learn how to develop a patient and family education program that meets the needs of your organization and its patients, and how to avoid Type I recommendations on these standards. **($67/copy, 136 pages #PFN)**

Performance Improvement: Winning Strategies for Quality and JCAHO Compliance

by Cynthia Barnard, MM, CPHQ, and Jodi Eisenberg, CMSC
Written by two health care quality and accreditation specialists whose hospital scored in the top 1% of hospitals nationally in a recent JCAHO survey, this book offers you a step-by-step approach to developing a strong PI program in your organization.

This book will help you to:
- prioritize your PI initiatives and ensure that you focus on issues that really matter;
- determine what you do and don't need to include in your PI plan and PI program;
- demystify performance measurement and assessment;
- conduct the required PI program self-assessment once all of your improvements have been made;

- understand the new ORYX initiative;
- understand what hospital leaders' PI responsibilities are and how to garner leadership's support of your PI program;
- prepare staff and leaders for the surveyors' PI questions;
- ensure that the hospital meets Joint Commission standards; and
- prepare for the key PI-related sessions of your JCAHO survey.

($87/copy, 197 pages #PIN)

Ready, Set, JCAHO! Questions, Games, and Other Strategies to Prepare Your Staff for Survey

by Candace J. Hamner, RN, MA

Ready, Set, JCAHO! was created to make your job easier. This book provides universal techniques for helping everyone be prepared and more at ease when survey day arrives. It presents simple, easy, and entertaining ways to disseminate essential information to staff throughout your organization. From quizzes and games to theme days and contests, *Ready, Set, JCAHO!* offers both traditional and non-traditional training approaches.
($97/copy, 274 pages #RSJN)

Restraint and Seclusion: Improving Practice and Conquering the JCAHO Standards, Second Edition

by Jack Zusman, MD

This book dissects and analyzes the JCAHO's standards relating to restraint and seclusion in clear, concise language. *Restraint and Seclusion* examines the pros and cons of restraint use, presents ideas for improving patient care in your organization, and discusses issues that relate specifically to seclusion. In addition, this book will enable you to

- understand when and why restraints should be used;
- reduce the risk of physical injury and minimize psychological and social harm to patients in restraint and seclusion;
- address legal risk, patient consent, and staff education; and
- create detailed policies and procedures using the samples provided.

($87/copy, 200 pages #RUMN)

Newsletters

Briefings on JCAHO

At over 3,700 hospitals nationwide, *Briefings on JCAHO* is the respected voice of authority for practical, independent guidance on succeeding in the accreditation process. Whether you're new to the survey game or are a seasoned professional, each issue offers quick reading and "how-to" advice on meeting JCAHO standards. For about $27 a month, you'll get tips and information that would otherwise cost you dearly in consulting fees and research. **($327/year [12 issues] #BOJ12)**

Medical Staff Briefing

This monthly publication is uniquely written for medical staff coordinators and physician leaders. From offering ideas on streamlining medical staff processes to developing physician leadership and improving credentialing and privileging, *Medical Staff Briefing* reports it all. While physician leaders get the assistance they need, medical staff services professionals get the support they need: fewer mistakes, better compliance, and improved relationships at all levels. **($327/year [12 issues] #MSB12)**

Respiratory Care Manager

Respiratory Care Manager, the first monthly newsletter written especially for managers in respiratory care, provides valuable information to help them succeed in their leadership functions. This newsletter is on the pulse of this ever-changing profession, bringing together the latest news and trends that impact the respiratory care manager's daily, on-the-job decisions. **($167/year [12 issues] #RCM12)**

Videos

Turning JCAHO Confusion into Confidence: How Every Employee Can Answer the JCAHO's Top Survey Questions

Geared for everyone from the CEO or nurse manager to an environmental service worker or registration clerk, *Turning JCAHO Confusion into Confidence* provides universal techniques for helping everyone in the hospital be better prepared and more at ease when survey day arrives. This 15-minute video and the accompanying training materials will teach your staff how to make a positive contribution to the hospital's survey, regardless of what role they play within the organization.
($295/tape, 15 min. #VTCC)